CLINICAL ENT

An Illustrated Textbook

Second Edition

CLINICAL ENT

An Illustrated Textbook

Second Edition

GERARD M. O'DONOGHUE, MCh, FRCS
Consultant ENT Surgeon University Hospital, Nottingham

ANTONY A. NARULA, MA, FRCS
Consultant ENT Surgeon, The Leicester Royal Infirmary, Leicester

GRANT J. BATES, BSc, FRCS
Consultant ENT Surgeon, Radcliffe Infirmary, Oxford

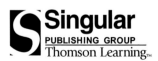

Singular
PUBLISHING GROUP
Thomson Learning

Singular Publishing Group
Thomson Learning
401 West A Street, Suite 325
San Diego, California 92101-7904

M W

Singular Publishing Group, Inc., publishes textbooks, clinical manuals, clinical reference books, journals, videos, and multimedia materials on speech-language pathology, audiology, otorhinolaryngology, special education, early childhood, aging, occupational therapy, physical therapy, rehabilitation, counseling, mental health, and voice. For your convenience, our entire catalog can be accessed on our website at *http://www.singpub.com.* Our mission to provide you with materials to meet the daily challenges of the ever-changing health care/educational environment will remain on course if we are in touch with you. In that spirit, we welcome your feedback on our products. Please telephone (**1-800-521-8545**), fax (**1-800-774-8398**), or e-mail (*singpub@singpub.com*) your comments and requests to us.

Typeset in 10/12 Palatino by Thompson Type
Printed in Canada by Transcontinental

Library of Congress Cataloging-in-Publication Data
O'Donoghue, Gerard M.
    Clinical ENT: an illustrated textbook/by Gerard M. O'Donoghue, Antony A. Narula, Grant J. Bates.—2nd ed.
      p. cm.
    Includes index.
    ISBN 1-56593-993-X (softcover: alk. paper)
    1. Otolaryngology.   I. Narula, Antony A.   II. Bates, Grant J.
III. Title.
    [DNLM: 1. Otorhinolaryngologic Diseases.   WV 140 026c 2000]
RF46.033   2000
617.5'1—dc21
DNLM/DLC
for Library of Congress   99-31868
                                                     CIP

11/21/02

Contents

....

PART I: THE EAR

PART II: THE NOSE AND SINUSES

PART III: THE LARYNX, HEAD, AND NECK

Foreword

···

Drs O'Donoghue, Narula, and Bates have succeeded in putting together a well written, concise, and eminently practical manual covering a broad spectrum of otolaryngologic diseases. Students seeking a comprehensive introduction to the field will appreciate its manageable size and utility both as a cover-to-cover introductory text as well as a terse reference source to individual topics of interest. Busy practitioners will value its practice-oriented approach to guide them in managing ENT common problems. This book is ideally suited for nonspecialists who seek to learn aspects of the field they might handle themselves. Guidelines are provided to help recognize when specialty referral is advisable. A particular strength of the book, as emphasized in its title, is the number and quality of its illustrations. An abundance of original illustrations, high resolution images (eg, CT and MRI scans), and clinical photographs emphasizing diagnostic clinical findings have been included. The numerous tables, which display key diagnostic points and therapeutic alternatives, are also most worthwhile.

In the outpatient practice of medicine, a remarkably high fraction of patients seen by primary care practitioners have problems referable to the head and neck region. Physicians who strive to develop well-rounded clinical capabilities in this regard would be well served by adding this up-to-date reference to their library.

Robert K. Jackler, MD
Professor of Otolaryngology and Neurological Surgery
University of California, San Francisco

Preface

···

The challenge the authors faced was this: How to convey the excitement of this bustling specialty to the contemporary medical student? The development that has characterized ENT in recent years is extremely impressive. Much has to be attributed to advances in sensory physiology with which our specialty is intimately linked. For instance, developments in auditory neurophysiology have revolutionized the assessment of inner ear disorders and paved the way for such important advances as cochlear implantation. The skull base, previously a surgical "no man's land," is now eminently accessible using microsurgical techniques. Endoscopic surgery has had a major impact on the understanding and treatment of nasal and sinus disorders and advanced the evaluation and surgery of the larynx and trachea. Better reconstructive techniques have become available to minimize the morbidity from major head and neck resections. The use of lasers and microvascular techniques has been especially valuable. Voice disorders, cosmetic surgery, sleep disturbance, and molecular biology are examples of other areas engaging much of the ENT surgeon's attention.

Care has been taken to cover the basics of ENT assessment and common clinical conditions are presented in a succinct manner, often illustrated by clinical photographs. Realizing that medical students too have their pressures, key points have been interspersed throughout the text to emphasize the essentials and help with the inevitable last minute revision! We also hope the book will help family practitioners, casualty officers, pediatricians, and the many physicians whose practice brings them to bear on that great temple of surprises—the head and neck.

Gerard O'Donoghue
Antony A. Narula
Grant J. Bates

Acknowledgments

···

The authors are indebted to the many colleagues and students who helped in the preparation of this book, especially those who courageously offered their criticism!

Many illustrations and photographs were generously loaned to us by our friends. The eminent French otologist Dr.Christian Deguine from Lille readily put his remarkable collection of tympanic membrane photographs at our disposal. *Merci infiniment Christian*. Mr. Michael Rothera, FRCS, Manchester, kindly provided Figures 8-17, 8-18,8-19, 9-5, and 9-6. We also wish to thank Mr. Andrew Freeland, FRCS, Oxford, and Oxford University Press (Fig 1-5), Dr. Steve Mason, Nottingham (Figs 3-5, 3-6, 6-4, 6-9, 8-2, and 8-3), and Dr. Julian McGlashen, Nottingham (Fig 28-9).

We are indebted to the Medical Illustration Departments at University Hospital Nottingham and the Leicester Royal Infirmary for their contributions.

A special word of thanks to Raphaële, Charlotte, Susan, and the children—without their understanding, patience, and sense of humor, we might have faltered in our mission.

PART ONE

The Ear

CHAPTER 1

Clinical Anatomy and Physiology

....

The ear is a sensory end organ serving the demands of hearing and balance.

THE EXTERNAL EAR

The external ear (Fig 1-1) helps collect and localize sound. It is formed by the pinna and external ear canal. The pinna is made of elastic cartilage covered by skin. The skin is tightly adherent to the perichondrium on the outer surface of the pinna. A hematoma

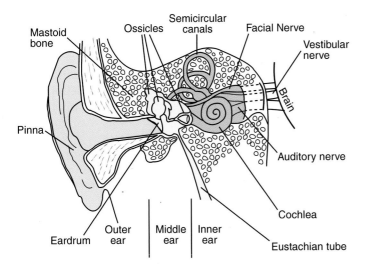

Fig 1-1 A coronal section through the ear. Sound is collected by the external ear, amplified by the middle ear, and converted into electrical impulses by the inner ear. Note that the facial nerve courses through the ear.

may detach the perichondrium and devascularize the cartilage. Deficiencies in the cartilage of the ear canal can facilitate the spread of infection and malignancy to the parotid and skull base.

In the adult, the external ear canal is between 2 and 3 cm in length. The outer one third is cartilaginous and the inner two thirds is bony. The ear canal is slightly curved and to allow

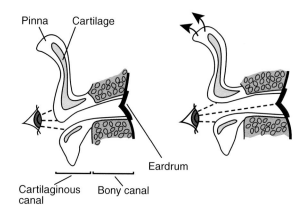

Fig 1-2 To inspect the tympanic membrane the ear canal must be straightened. This is done by gently retracting the pinna upward and backward.

Pinna Cartilage

Eardrum

Cartilaginous canal Bony canal

inspection must be straightened by gently retracting the pinna upward and backward (Fig 1-2).

The inner two thirds of the ear canal is lined by highly specialized stratified squamous epithelium, which is devoid of hair follicles and does not desquamate. This skin has the property, unique in the body, of lateral migration. This is an active process, starting at the eardrum, and progresses at the rate of about 100 μm per day. This "conveyor belt" keeps the ear canal clean, which is essential for efficient air conduction. Attempts by patients to clean their ears with cotton swabs only serve to push wax and debris further down the ear canal and such practices should be discouraged. The skin of the outer third of the ear canal is identical to skin elsewhere on the body.

Wax is formed by ceruminous glands in the outer portion of the ear canal. It prevents the ingress of particulate matter into the ear and also has a surface immunoprotective function. It only needs to be removed if it becomes impacted (usually in people who clean their ears). The oily property of this wax was used by ancient monks to illuminate their manuscripts!

The *lymphatics* of the external ear drain to the retroauricular, parotid, retropharyngeal, and upper deep cervical lymph nodes. These may become enlarged and tender in infections or neoplasms of the external ear.

THE MIDDLE EAR

The *tympanic membrane* (Figs 1-3 and 1-4) or eardrum separates the external and middle ears. It has a dense fibrous middle layer and an inner layer lined by middle ear mucosa. Its small upper portion, above the lateral process, is called the *pars flaccida*, because its middle fibrous layer is relatively lax. The lower portion is called the *pars tensa* and is the part of the drum responsive to sound. In health it is virtually transparent and exhibits a *light reflex* on otoscopic examination (this is due to its slightly conical

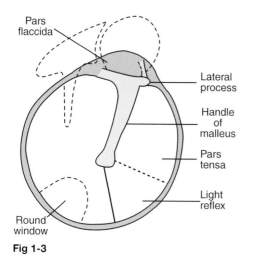

Pars flaccida
Lateral process
Handle of malleus
Pars tensa
Light reflex
Round window

Fig 1-3

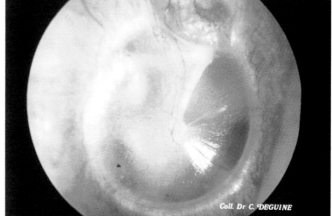

Coll. Dr C. DEGUINE

Fig 1-4

shape). The malleus handle can be seen embedded in the ear drum. The tympanic membrane measures about 1 cm in diameter and its center is called the umbo.

The middle ear is an air-containing space bounded laterally by the tympanic membrane and medially by the basal turn of the cochlea, called the promontory. Its capacity is about 1 cm³. It contains a chain of three bones or ossicles: the malleus, which is the largest and is embedded in the tympanic membrane; the incus, in the middle; and the stapes, lying in contact with the inner ear at the oval window. The incus is delicately poised and is the ossicle most likely to be dislocated following head injury. Tiny muscles attach to the malleus and stapes to dampen vibration and protect the inner ear from excessive noise.

The middle ear is important because infection can spread through it to vital structures only a few millimeters away. Superiorly lies the middle cranial fossa (containing the temporal lobe). Posteriorly, the mastoid air cells are adjacent to the posterior fossa (containing the cerebellum) and the lateral (sigmoid) sinus. Medially, the lateral semicircular canal can be eroded by chronic suppuration which allows bacteria access to the inner ear. The *facial nerve* runs through the middle ear and can also be damaged by inflammatory processes.

The eustachian tube connects the middle ear to the nasopharynx. Oxygen is constantly absorbed by the mucosa of the middle ear, resulting in a negative middle ear pressure. The eustachian tube is responsible for the equalization of pressure between the middle ear and the outside world. The tube is normally closed but has muscles attached to it which open the tube on swallowing or yawning. Its function is particularly important during flying and diving to enable rapid equalization of pressure on both sides of the tympanic membrane. The tube undergoes major structural changes during development: In infancy it is short and

Fig 1-3 The normal tympanic membrane (left). The conical shape of the membrane causes the light reflex. Note the position of the lateral process and handle of malleus. Deep to the membrane, the long process of incus and round window niche can sometimes be seen. The pars flaccida lies above the lateral process.

Fig 1-4 Normal tympanic membrane (right). Compare this with Fig 1-3. Note its semitransparent quality. The silhouette of the long process of incus and round window niche can just be appreciated through the intact membrane.

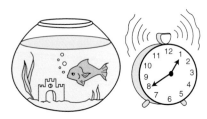

Fig 1-5 The goldfish is unperturbed by the alarm clock as most of the airborne sound is reflected at the air-water interface. Without the amplifying action of the middle ear in man, almost all of the incident sound energy would be reflected away from the inner ear.

almost horizontal but during childhood it becomes elongated, with a slight downward angulation. The relative immaturity of the tube contributes to the high prevalence of childhood middle ear disease.

The inner ear structures are immersed in fluid. The transmission of sound energy from air (ie, as in the middle ear) to a fluid medium results in substantial loss of sound energy (Fig 1-5). To overcome this, the middle ear needs to amplify sound. This is achieved by virtue of the fact that the surface area of the tympanic membrane is 20 times that of the oval window. Furthermore, the shape of the chain of ossicles is such as to confer a mechanical advantage for sound transmission.

THE INNER EAR

The inner ear comprises the cochlea, vestibular labyrinth, and their central connections. These delicate structures are embedded in dense bone called the otic capsule. The facial nerve courses through the inner ear.

The Cochlea

The cochlea is a minute spiral of 2½ turns. Within this spiral, perilymph and endolymph are partitioned by the thinnest of membranes. Biochemically, the inner ear fluids are quite different, with endolymph having a high concentration of potassium (ie, 144 mEq/L, similar to intracellular fluid) and perilymph being high in sodium (Fig 1-6). The maintenance of these ionic concentrations is an active process effected by sodium and potassium pumps.

To understand how this complex structure works, it is best to unravel its spiral arrangement (Fig 1-7). The endolymphatic compartment containing the sensory epithelium is completely surrounded by perilymph. Each compression caused by the stapes

Fig 1-6 The biochemical concentrations of inner ear fluids. Cerebrospinal fluid is similar to perilymph with which it communicates. Endolymph has a high potassium concentration similar to intracellular fluid.

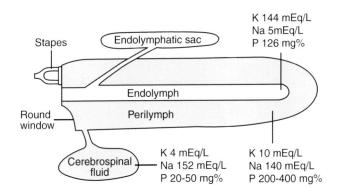

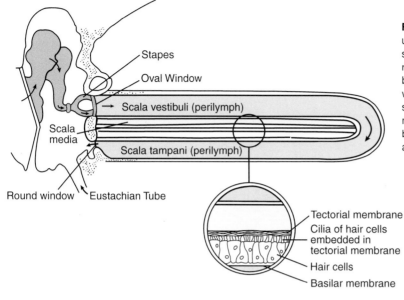

Fig 1-7 The spiral of the cochlea is undone. Each compression at the stapes causes a rarefaction at the round window (the inner ear fluid being incompressible). A travelling wave is generated, which maximally stimulates certain parts of the basilar membrane: high frequencies at the base of the cochlea, low frequencies at the apex.

footplate results in a corresponding rarefaction of the round window membrane. A travelling wave is generated which causes maximum resonance in the particular portion of the basilar membrane that roughly corresponds to the particular stimulus frequency. The lower frequencies register in the apical turn, the higher frequencies in the basal turn. Although minute, the cochlea accommodates an intensity range of 1 000 000:1. For reasons of practicality, this vast range is compressed into a logarithmic decibel scale of 0 to 120 dB (Fig 1-8). The frequency range of the human ear is from 20 to 20 000 Hz.

The basic physiological unit in the cochlea is the *hair cell* (Fig 1-9). There are about 15 000 such cells in the human ear. They are arranged in rows of inner and outer cells. The hair cells act as mechano-electric transducers converting the acoustic signal into an electrical impulse (Fig 1-10). The slightest displacement of the hairs causes rapid ionic shifts to occur, with depolarization of the cell followed by an immediate return to the resting potential. This electrical impulse is carried from hair cell to neuron by release of a chemical neurotransmitter. Such is the sensitivity of hair cells that they respond within a few millionths of a second to movements of 100 picometers, which is no more than the diameter of an atom!

The auditory nerve carries impulses to the cochlear nuclei in the brain stem. Each nerve fiber is "tuned" to respond best to a particular frequency, giving it a characteristic "tuning" curve. Most fibers cross to the opposite side of the brain stem and travel to the lateral lemniscus and medial geniculate body. From there, the fibers travel to the auditory cortex which is located in the superior temporal gyrus of the cerebral cortex.

	dB	
Painful	140	firearms
	130	jackhammer
	120	jet plane takeoff
Extremely loud	110	rock music
	100	chain saw
	90	lawnmower
Very loud	80	alarm clock
	70	busy traffic
	60	conversation
Moderate	50	
	40	quiet room
Faint	30	whisper

Fig 1-8 The decibel scale. A whisper is about 20 dB, conversational voice about 60 dB, and a jet aircraft 120 dB. The scale is logarithmic to accommodate the vast intensity range of the human ear.

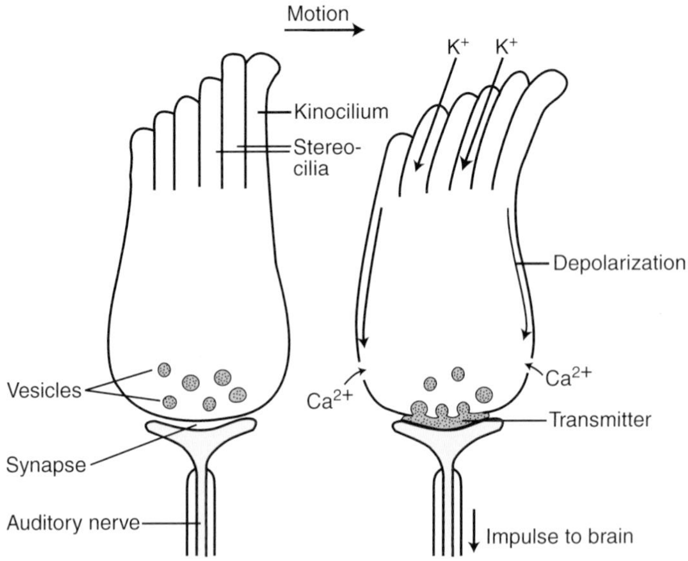

Fig 1-9 A hair cell. The slightest motion (eg, the diameter of a hydrogen atom!) of the hairs causes rapid depolarization of the cell. This results in the release of an unknown neurotransmitter which excites the auditory neuron. The impulse is then carried along the auditory nerve.

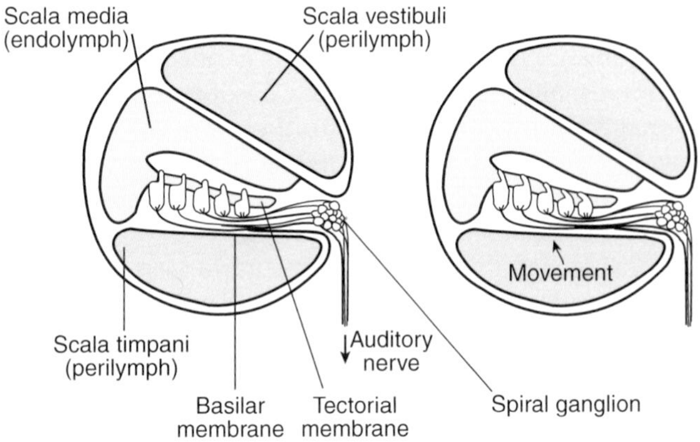

Fig 1-10 Movement of the basilar membrane in response to sound results in a shearing of the hair cells which are embedded in the tectorial membrane. Impulses generated in this way are then carried via the auditory nerve.

The Vestibular Labyrinth

This comprises the semicircular canals, the utricle, saccule, and their central connections. The three semicircular canals (horizontal, superior, and posterior) are arranged in the 3 planes of space at right angles to each other.

Like the auditory system, the vestibular end organ responds to hair cell movement (Fig 1-11). In the lateral canals, the hair cells are embedded in a gelatinous cupula and are sheared during angular movements of the head. In the utricle and saccule, the hair cells are embedded in an otoconial membrane containing particles of calcium carbonate. These respond to changes in linear acceleration and the pull of gravity. Impulses are carried centrally by the vestibular nerve. The major connections of the vestibular system are to the spinal cord, cerebellum, and external ocular muscles.

The maintenance of balance is dependent not only on the integrity of the vestibular apparatus but also on input from proprioceptive and visual systems and the cerebellum.

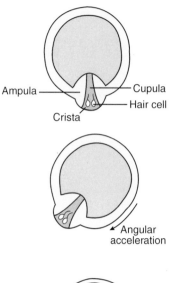

> **Key Point:**
> The hair cells of the inner ear act by converting sound and acceleration into electrical energy which excites the auditory and vestibular nerves.

SENSORY INNERVATION OF THE EAR

The ear has a rich and diverse supply of sensory nerves, which explains why referred pain to the ear is a frequent finding in clinical practice:

External Ear

Great auricular (C2 and C3), Lesser occipital (C2)
Auriculo temporal (Cranial nerve V)
Sensory branch of facial (Cranial nerve VII)
Vagus (Cranial nerve X)

Middle Ear

Glossopharyngeal (Cranial nerve IX)

Inner Ear

No somatic sensory innervation

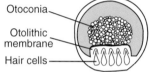

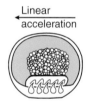

Referred otalgia may come from the normal area of distribution of any of these nerves.

> **Key Point:**
> Referred pain to the ear may come from many structures in the head and neck (eg, a sore throat or impacted wisdom tooth). Always examine the oral cavity and pharynx to exclude infection or tumor.

Fig 1-11 Angular and linear acceleration cause shearing of hair cells in the semicircular canals, utricle, and saccule. Impulses generated in this way are carried by the vestibular nerve to the cerebellum, spinal cord, and the nuclei of the ocular muscles.

CHAPTER 2

History and Examination

The ear is a superficial structure on the side of the head and can be readily inspected. It is disappointing to find that examination is so often inadequate or not undertaken at all. One should not be deterred by the mystique of the head mirror or microscope!

HISTORY

Diseases of the ear can only express themselves in a very limited number of ways (Table 2-1).

Table 2-1. The Five Principal Symptoms of Ear Disease

1. Earache
2. Deafness
3. Discharge
4. Tinnitus
5. Vertigo

Earache (Otalgia)

The ear has a rich sensory innervation (p9). Earache usually indicates an inflammatory process in the external or middle ear. The onset of the pain, its duration, severity, aggravating and relieving factors, as well as the presence of any associated symptoms, will need to be determined. The quantity of analgesics taken by the patient and the amount of time lost from school or work are useful pointers to the severity of the pain. Referred pain may come from many head and neck structures (wisdom teeth, jaw joint, floor of mouth, tonsil, cervical spine, etc).

Deafness

There are four key questions:

Was the onset sudden or gradual? Sudden hearing loss may occur in a number of circumstances, for example following barotrauma (flying or diving), upper respiratory infection, exposure to excessive noise, drug administration (eg, gentamicin), or head injury.

Is it unilateral or bilateral? Remember that unilateral losses are more likely to have a specific underlying cause. Deafness due to aging or noise exposure is not unilateral. The commonest presenting symptom of an acoustic neuroma is unilateral hearing loss, which is often very slight and insidious. Bilateral hearing loss may have a genetic basis or be due to systemic disease.

Is the loss progressive, fluctuating, or improving? Deafness due to aging or continued noise exposure is often progressive. Ménière's disease and serous otitis media typically present with fluctuating hearing loss. An acute middle ear effusion following an upper respiratory infection usually shows steady improvement.

What is the hearing like in group conversation? Generally, patients with conductive hearing loss manage reasonably well in group conversation. Patients with sensorineural hearing loss have poor speech discrimination in noise and usually admit to doing better in one-to-one conversation. This question will also help assess the impact of the hearing impairment on the patient's ability to communicate in everyday life.

Discharge (Otorrhea)

- Diseases of the external ear produce a scanty discharge.

- Copious discharge is always from the middle ear.

- Smelly discharge suggests cholesteatoma.

- Bloody discharge follows ear canal trauma, severe acute infection or tumor.

- Watery discharge can be cerebrospinal fluid.

> **Key Point:**
> Mucoid discharge must come from the middle ear as there are no mucous glands in the external ear.

Tinnitus

Tinnitus is the name given to the symptom of noises in the head or ears. Enquiry should be made about the circumstances of onset, the type of noise, its location, duration, and intensity. Tinnitus that is pulsatile may be due to vascular abnormality or tumor. Often the noises are most troublesome at night when the patient is trying to get to sleep. This is due to the absence of background noise. Tinnitus is a common accompaniment of hearing impairment from any cause.

Vertigo

This term describes the hallucination of movement of the environment about the patient or of the patient in relation to the environment. It is *not* synonymous with dizziness. Vertigo is a symptom of a disorder of the peripheral labyrinth or of the central vestibular pathways. The issues to determine in relation to vertigo are as follows:

Onset

If the symptom started following barotrauma (flying or diving), acoustic trauma, or head injury, rupture of an inner ear membrane

Key Points:

1. A detailed history is the most important requirement for making a correct diagnosis in a dizzy patient.

2. Vertigo is a specific symptom describing a hallucination of movement. It must be differentiated from dizziness.

3. In a patient with vertigo the most important diagnostic pointers are the duration of attacks and the presence or absence of auditory or neurological symptoms.

4. Central causes of vertigo will generally have associated neurological symptoms or signs.

(perilymph fistula, p50) should be considered. Acute fulminant vertigo without hearing loss in an otherwise healthy young adult is likely to be due to vestibular neuronitis. If the symptom lasts a few seconds on adopting a sudden change of posture without any hearing loss, consider benign positional vertigo (BPV). Dysequilibrium (rather than vertigo) lasting over many years may have a psychogenic basis.

Duration

In Ménière's disease, the vertigo lasts between half an hour and 8 to 10 hours. In BPV, the vertigo lasts for only a few seconds. In vestibular neuronitis, the duration is 2 to 3 days.

Associated Symptoms

The presence of auditory symptoms strongly supports a peripheral labyrinthine cause and should always be asked about. Nausea and vomiting, as in sea sickness, are typical accompaniments of labyrinthine vertigo. Central causes of vertigo (eg, vertebrobasilar insufficiency, multiple sclerosis) are associated with other neurological symptoms (eg, dysarthria, visual disturbance) and are not typically accompanied by auditory symptoms. Limitation of neck movement may indicate cervical vertigo.

EXAMINATION INSTRUMENTS

The instruments required for examination of the ear are shown in Fig 2-1.

Technique

Position

The examination is best performed when the examiner and the patient are seated comfortably (Fig 2-2). It is distressing to see a patient seated while the physician stands, screwing his spinal column into contortions and perilously grasping an otoscope (Fig 2-3). This is likely to be both unproductive and hazardous. Therefore, sit comfortably at the patient's level.

Inspection

Inspect the pinna. Having done so, bend it forward and look behind the ear (Fig 2-4). This may reveal the scarring of previous surgery, a swelling (which is often inflammatory), or the ulceration typical of malignancy. Bat ears is the term given to abnormally protuberant ears. Deformity of the pinna may be a clue to congenital hearing loss.

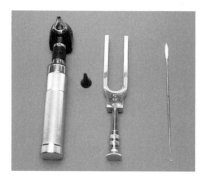

Fig 2-1 Tools of the trade! From left to right: a fiberoptic otoscope with disposable speculae; a tuning fork (512 Hz); a Jobson Horne probe (one end can act as a cotton wool carrier and the other is used for wax removal).

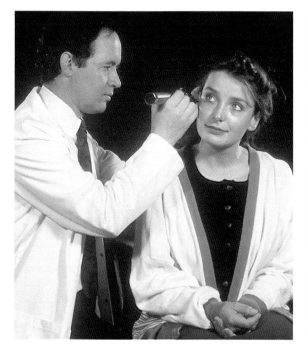

Fig 2-2 When patient and examiner are at the same level, the examination is greatly facilitated.

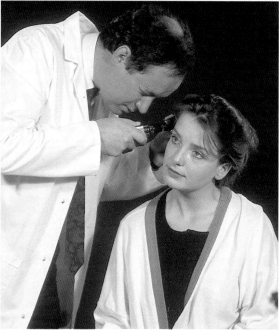

Fig 2-3 This awkward posture has nothing to recommend it. Note the poor control over the otoscope, which is being held like a dagger.

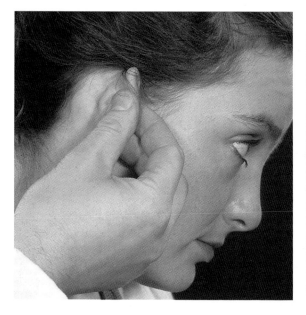

Fig 2-4 This maneuver should be done in every case. It is surprising what the pinna can hide—scars, swellings due to infection, or tumors.

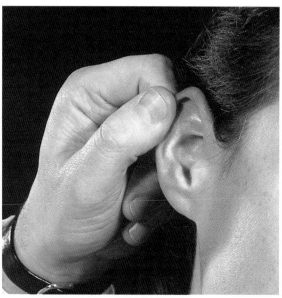

Fig 2-5 Retracting the pinna upward and backward straightens the external ear canal and is a prerequisite for inspecting the tympanic membrane.

Otoscopy

Hold the otoscope like an artist holds a brush—delicately but with full control. *Gently* retract the pinna to straighten the ear canal (Fig 2-5)—bear in mind that in inflammatory conditions of the ear this movement alone can be painful. Watch the patient's facial expression—if there are signs of grimacing, proceed only with the greatest caution. Always steady the hand that holds the instrument on the patient's cheek (Figs 2-6 and 2-7). This is essential to prevent injury to the external ear should the patient suddenly jolt. If wax is present, it will need removal by syringing.

Once the ear canal has been cleared, it is essential to examine the entire tympanic membane (Figs 2-8 and 2-9). There is a tendency to satisfy oneself with seeing the pars tensa but the pars flaccida is more often the seat of destructive ear disease. To examine the pars flaccida, direct the light at the most superior aspect of the ear drum while tilting the patient's head away.

The mobility of the ear drum can be determined by using the pneumatic attachment on the otoscope (see Fig 2-1), provided the speculum is a snug fit for the ear canal.

Tuning Forks

Tuning fork testing must be included in the assessment. The tests demand good technique and a basic understanding of air and bone conduction. The tests most commonly employed are the Rinne and Weber tests.

The Rinne Test. This compares hearing through air and bone conduction. Normally, we hear by air conduction which is more efficient than hearing through bone. To do the test, briefly explain to the patient that you are going to place a tuning fork behind and then in front of the ear and that you will want to know in which position the fork sounds loudest. Strike the tuning fork (512 Hz) against your elbow or kneecap (not on the floor or table-top—this produces undesirable overtones). Then steady the patient's head with one hand and apply the base of the tuning fork firmly to the patient's mastoid bone for at least 2 to 3 seconds, ie, sufficient time for the patient to make a mental note of the intensity of the stimulus (Fig 2-10). Then bring the tuning fork around to the external ear canal (Fig 2-11) and again allow a few seconds for the patient to make a judgment. In a normal patient or in a patient with sensorineural hearing loss, the Rinne test is positive, ie, loudest in front of the ear. The Rinne test is said to be negative when the fork sounds loudest behind the ear. This is typical of conductive hearing loss greater than 20 dB.

A *false negative* Rinne test can be a pitfall for the unwary. If a patient has no cochlear function on one side, the Rinne test will be negative because the good ear (and *not* the test ear) is picking up

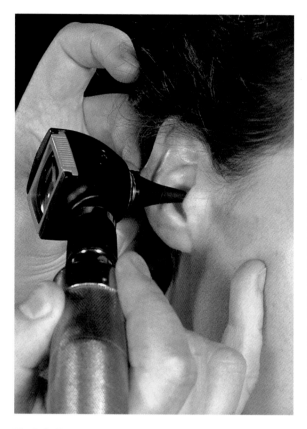

Fig 2-6 Always have control over any instrument (otoscope, wax hook, cotton wool carrier, etc) entering the external ear. The little finger resting on the cheek is the best "early warning" system. This is the arrangement for the right ear.

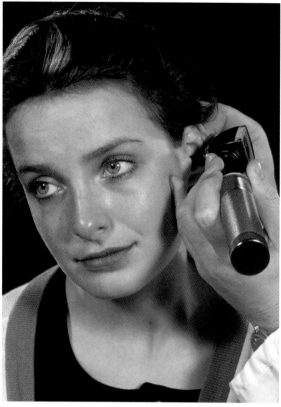

Fig 2-7 Examination of the left ear needs a change of hands.

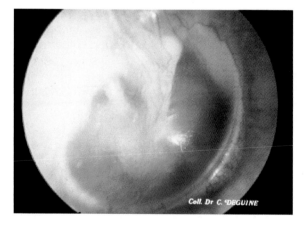

Fig 2-8 Normal tympanic membrane (right). Note its semitransparent quality. The silhouette of the long process of incus and round window niche can be appreciated through the intact membrane.

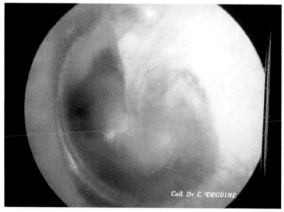

Fig 2-9 Normal tympanic membrane (left). Compare the landmarks on the right (Fig 2-8) and left ear drums. The lateral process of the malleus always points anteriorly.

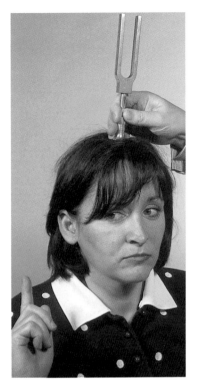

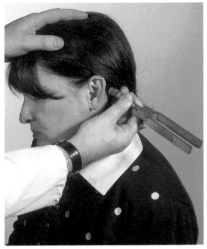

Fig 2-10 The Rinne test—bone conduction. To establish good bone contact, first steady the patient's head with one hand and then firmly apply the tuning fork to the mastoid bone.

Fig 2-11 The Rinne test—air conduction. When bringing the tuning fork to the "front," ensure the tines are parallel to the external ear canal.

Fig 2-12 The Weber test. Place the tuning fork firmly on a bony point in the midline (vertex, bridge of nose, incisor teeth). Weber to the left: the patient may rotate the eyes to the left or point to the left ear. This happens typically with a right conductive hearing loss.

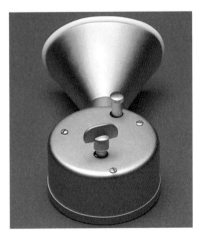

Fig 2-13 A Barany noise box used for masking the nontest ear.

the sound by means of bone conduction. To avoid this happening, the nontest ear must be masked ("kept busy") during testing, ie, by massaging the tragus. The Weber test will usually save the day by being referred to the only hearing ear.

The Weber Test. In this test the tuning fork is placed in the midline (usually at the vertex or on the bridge of the nose) and the patient is asked to indicate in which ear, if any, the noise sounds loudest. Again, explain the procedure to the patient before you proceed with the test. Normally, the sound is perceived in the midline. If one ear has a sensorineural deficit, the sound lateralizes to the better cochlea. If a conductive loss is present on one side, the tuning fork lateralizes to the side of the conductive loss (Fig 2-12).

Conversational Testing

Conversational testing offers a useful guide to the level of hearing impairment. It must be done without giving the patient any visual clues such as the examiner's lip movements. In many situations, the nontest ear will need to be prevented from hearing. This is done by using a noise box (Fig 2-13) or by simply massaging the tragus of the nontest ear while simultaneously asking the

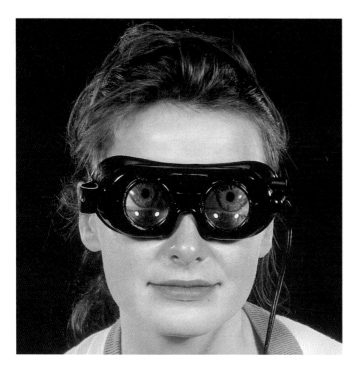

Fig 2-14 Frenzel's glasses. These remove optic fixation by having +20 diopter lenses—try them on yourself! They magnify the eyeball and make eye movements much easier to define. Removing optic fixation makes nystagmus from inner ear disease much more obvious.

patient to repeat words or numbers spoken near the ear under test. To a rough approximation, a whisper is about 30 decibels; a softly spoken voice is about 50 decibels.

Nystagmus

Nystagmus is involuntary oscillatory movement of the eyes. It can be a normal phenomenon. If you sit opposite someone who is looking out of the window in a fast moving train you will observe the eyes flicker every few seconds. This nystagmus has 2 components: a quick component due to central compensation and a slow phase which is due to peripheral mechanisms. By convention, the direction of a nystagmus is the direction of the fast component. Peripheral nystagmus tends to be suppressed by optic fixation and hence is enhanced in darkness or by wearing Frenzel's glasses (Fig 2-14). These glasses have +20 diopter lenses, which allow the examiner a magnified view of the eye movements but prevent the patient from using optic fixation.

Horizontal jerk nystagmus is typical of peripheral labyrinthine disorders. This has a slow movement in one direction followed by a quick jerk in the opposite direction. Nystagmus due to central disorders, eg, multiple sclerosis or brain stem compression, tends to be much more complex and often bizarre.

Nystagmus induced by positional testing is a useful test in patients with benign positional vertigo. The patient is asked to sit on

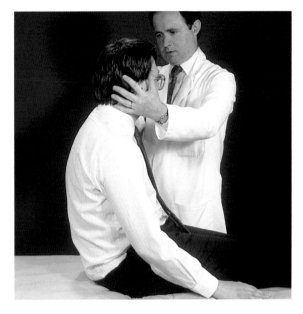

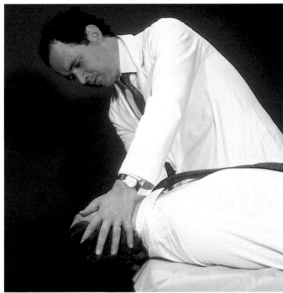

Fig 2-15 Positional testing. The starting position must be such as to allow the patient's head to be dropped below the horizontal when the patient is thrust backwards (Fig 2-16).

Fig 2-16 Positional testing. Note that the head is below the level of the couch and rotated to one side. The patient's eyes should be open to observe nystagmus. The test should not be done in patients with restricted neck mobility.

an examining couch and the head is thrust suddenly backwards to just below the level of the couch (Figs 2-15 and 2-16). In benign positional vertigo, nystagmus is induced when the affected ear is lowermost. The nystagmus comes on after a second or so and lasts for several seconds. It is of a rotatory type and is fatiguable, ie, it disappears with repeated testing. The test is not a way to win friends but is clinically very useful!

Fistula Test

This is performed by raising and lowering the pressure in the external ear (usually with a pneumatic otoscope or by a pumping action on the tragus). The test is said to be positive if the maneuver induces nystagmus and vertigo. This typically occurs if an inner ear membrane ruptures following excessive pressure changes during flying or diving (barotrauma). It also occurs when the labyrinth is eroded by cholesteatoma.

Facial Nerve

The facial nerve is motor to the facial muscles and to the stapedius muscle in the middle ear. Always check facial nerve

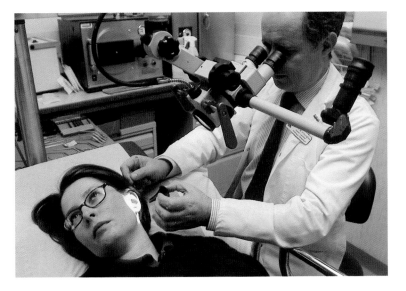

Fig 2-17 Examination under the microscope (EUM). This allows inspection under magnification of the external ear, middle ear, or mastoid cavity. Ears containing debris or wax can be suction cleaned under a microscope. A myringotomy (drainage of fluid from the middle ear) can be performed in clinic using this technique.

function in diseases of the ear. Usually the diagnosis is obvious but a subtle weakness (see Figs 7-4 and 7-7) or a bilateral paralysis (see Figs 7-2 and 7-3) can easily escape detection.

Examination Under the Microscope (EUM)

This is standard procedure in all ENT departments (Fig 2-17). A speculum is placed in the external ear canal and the pinna is retracted. Using this technique, ears can be dewaxed, foreign bodies removed, and minor surgery (eg, myringotomy or grommet insertion) can be undertaken. A valuable adjunct is the use of suction to remove debris from an ear.

Key Points:

1. Conductive hearing losses are due to disorders of the external or middle ear.

2. Sensorineural hearing losses are due to disorders of the cochlea or of the auditory nerve.

3. Tuning fork tests can determine whether a hearing loss is conductive or sensorineural and should always be performed. They will not indicate the level of hearing loss.

4. The Rinne test will not become negative until a conductive hearing loss is in excess of 20 decibels.

The main steps in the examination of the ear are summarized in Table 2-2.

Table 2-2. ENT: History-Taking and Examination

Ear	Nose	Throat
History		
Earache, irritation	Obstruction	Hoarseness
Deafness	Rhinorrhea/postnasal drip	Dysphagia
Discharge	Allergy/hay fever	Stridor
Tinnitus	Facial pain	Lump in the neck
Vertigo	Epistaxis	Sleep disturbance
	Sense of smell	
	Appearance	
Children:		
Speech/language		
Past History		
Barotrauma	Trauma	Cigarette smoking
Acoustic trauma	Medications	Alcohol
Head injury	Prescribed	
	Nonprescribed	
Ototoxics		
Family history	Previous surgery	
Previous ear surgery		
Examination		
Pinna	Shape	Mouth
Mastoid	Septum	(palates, gums,
		teeth, tonsils)
Ear canal	Turbinates	Neck
Eardrum (esp. attic)	Airway	Larynx refer to ENT
Tuning forks	Mucopus	
Conversational test	Facial tenderness	
Nystagmus	Facial sensation	
Facial nerve	Facial swelling	

CHAPTER 3

Investigation of Auditory, Vestibular, and Facial Nerve Function

....

PURE TONE AUDIOMETRY

Pure tone audiometry is the test of auditory function most frequently undertaken. It is best performed in a soundproof booth (Fig 3-1). The test is dependent on patient cooperation and it is important that time is spent explaining to the patient what is involved. The patient wears headphones through which pure tones are presented to each ear in turn. The patient is asked to respond to sounds of decreasing intensity across the frequency range. Both air conduction and bone conduction can be tested (Fig 3-2). Bone conduction is a measure of cochlear function.

Acoustic separation of the ears can be a very difficult task. When testing visual acuity, the tester can simply occlude the eye

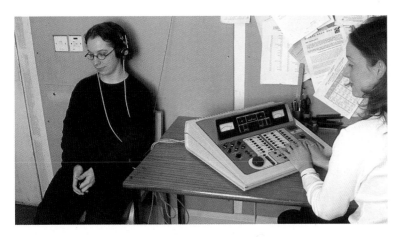

Fig 3-1 Pure tone audiometry being carried out in a soundproof booth. Sounds of decreasing intensity are presented and the patient is asked to press a trigger each time he hears a sound. No visual or temporal cues must be given to the patient about the sounds.

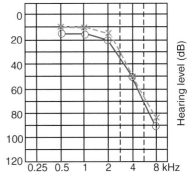

Fig 3-2 Pure tone audiogram. The zero decibel line represents the normal threshold. Hearing deficits are recorded on the vertical axis below this line. The low frequencies are on the horizontal axis. Agreed symbols are used for right and left ears and for air and bone conduction.

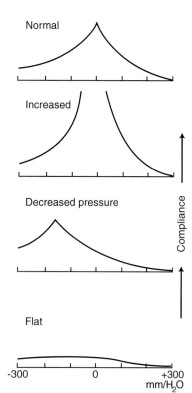

Normal

Increased

Decreased pressure

Compliance

Flat

-300   0   +300
                    mm/H$_2$O

Fig 3-3 The four most common types of tympanograms: *normal, increased compliance, decreased compliance,* and *flat.*

which is not being tested—this cannot be done so readily for hearing. The nontest ear must be masked ("kept busy") by applying a noise of appropriate intensity.

SPEECH AUDIOMETRY

In this test the patient is presented with phonetically balanced words and is scored on the number of correct responses.

TYMPANOMETRY

Tympanometry is a technique used extensively in clinical practice. It is based on the fact that the pressure in the external ear can be raised or lowered, thus stiffening the eardrum. A tympanometer presents a low-frequency sound to the ear and measures the sound energy reflected from the eardrum. The eardrum is most "floppy" when the pressure on both sides of it is equal. If fluid is present in the middle ear, the eardrum is unresponsive to changes in pressure of the external ear canal and a "flat" tracing is observed.

The 4 most common types of tympanogram are shown in Figure 3-3. *Normal:* occurs when pressures on both sides of the drum are equal at 0 on the pressure scale. *Increased:* occurs when the ear drum is "floppy" (thin scars, ossicular chain disrupted). *Decreased pressure:* occurs when the pressure in the middle ear is negative relative to the external ear (eg, eustachian tube dysfunction). *Flat:* occurs in middle ear effusions and is due to the fact that the fluid in the middle ear is incompressible.

Tympanometry is most useful in screening children for otitis media with effusion. The equipment is affordable in general practice.

STAPEDIAL REFLEXES

The stapedius muscle contracts in response to sound. This contraction stiffens the ossicular chain. This change in stiffness is readily detectable by measuring the resistance of the ossicular chain to sound transmission. In otosclerosis, a condition where the stapes bone is fixed, the stapedial reflex is absent. Scarring in the middle ear, caused by otitis media, can also result in loss of the reflex.

ELECTRIC RESPONSE AUDIOMETRY

Electric response audiometry is commonly used to assess the integrity of the cochlea and the central auditory pathways. Impulses originate in the cochlea and are carried by auditory nerve fibers to a number of relay stations in the brain stem before reaching the auditory cortex. By means of surface recording electrodes on the head and computer averaging techniques it is possible to study the response of the auditory pathways to sound.

If a single discrete sound is presented to the auditory system, the electrical response to it will be "drowned" by background activity from the brain (EEG) and muscles. If, however, thousands of time-locked discrete sounds are presented (rather like machine-gun fire), the electrical responses they generate can be added up to give a recognizable tracing. The background electrical activity in the brain, being random, will then cancel out. No anesthesia is generally required—the patient can even nod off to sleep during the study! There are 3 different types of electric responses in common usage :

1. *Electrocochleography (ECochG)*: This measures physiological events in the cochlea in response to sound (Fig 3-4). In Ménière's disease, specific changes are seen because the excess of fluid interferes with the mechanical properties of the membranes in the cochlea.

2. *Auditory Brainstem Responses (ABR)*: This resembles a nerve conduction study. The time taken for an impulse to get from the cochlea and through to the brain stem is measured. This time is prolonged by acoustic neuromas, even when they are tiny. Hence the role of this investigation in screening patients for these tumors (Fig 3-5). The test can be used as an objective hearing test in babies and young children.

   Neither of these 2 tests provides frequency specific information as in each case a broad bandwidth stimulus is used.

3. *Auditory Cortical Responses*: This technique measures the electrical activity in the auditory cortex in response to sounds of

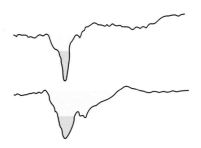

Fig 3-4 A normal electrocochleogram (above). Note the changes typical of an excess of fluid in the endolymph compartment, as occurs in Ménière's disease (below).

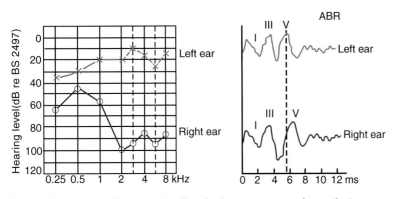

Fig 3-5 Pure tone audiogram and auditory brainstem responses in a patient with a right-sided acoustic neuroma. The hearing is normal in the left ear as is the I–V latency (broken vertical line represents upper limit of normal). On the right side, there is high frequency hearing loss and the I–V latency is prolonged. (*Note*: Wave I—distal cochlear nerve, Wave III—cochlear nuclei, and Wave V—tracts and nuclei of the lateral lemniscus).

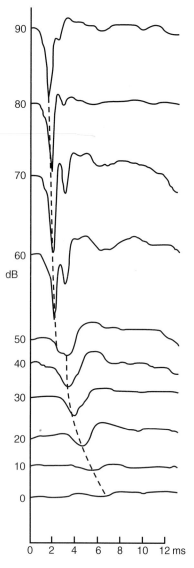

Fig 3-6 Auditory cortical responses in a normal ear. Note the waveforms can be traced from 90 dB almost to 0 dB.

different frequencies (Fig 3-6). The responses are particularly useful when assessing hearing in those patients who are either unable or unwilling to perform conventional audiometry. Thus, it is particularly useful in patients who may be exaggerating a hearing deficit in the pursuit of compensation.

OTOACOUSTIC EMISSIONS

Hair cells in the inner ear actually make sounds, called emissions, which can be detected by placing a highly sensitive microphone in the ear canal. As emisssions are exquisitely sensitive to disturbances of cochlear function, they are absent in patients with even mild hearing impairments. They thus have a pivotal role in the screening of neonates for sensorineural hearing loss. Emissions offer a lowcost, sensitive, and noninvasive means of undertaking universal neonatal hearing screening.

CALORIC AND ROTATION TESTING

The function of the semicircular canals is assessed by observing the effect on the system of warm and cold water stimulation. The vestibular nuclei have direct connections with the oculomotor nuclei. In the test, cold (30°C) and warm (44°C) water are introduced alternately into the external ear. This sets up convection currents in the lateral semicircular canals, which stimulate the vestibular system, producing nystagmus (involuntary eye movements). On cold water stimulation, the direction of the nystagmus (ie, that of the fast component) is to the opposite side, while warm water induces a nystagmus to the same side (the mnemonic COWS—Cold Opposite, Warm Sáme is helpful). The duration of the nystagmus is measured and the responses from left and right sides are compared.

The lateral semicircular canals can also be stimulated by rotating the patient while maintaining the rotational axis at horizontal. This simulates the natural stimulus to the canals. For caloric testing, the horizontal eye movements that result are monitored.

DYNAMIC POSTUROGRAPHY

Dynamic posturography represents a considerable advance in the investigation and rehabilitation of patients with chronic or intermittent balance disturbance. In these tests, the ability of patients to maintain posture in a variety of test situations is studied on specially designed platforms using computer-driven protocols. The findings can form the basis for designing more effective strategies for safe physical rehabilitation programs, especially for elderly patients.

ELECTRONYSTAGMOGRAPHY

This technique allows the eye movements that characterize nystagmus to be recorded graphically. It uses the fact that the eye is a rotating dipole, the retina being negative relative to the cornea. Recording electrodes are placed adjacent to the orbit and can record eye movements even when the eyes are closed (ie, with removal of optic fixation).

ELECTRONEURONOGRAPHY (ENoG)

This is used in the assessment of patients with facial paralysis. The facial nerve is electrically stimulated by placing electrodes on the skin above its exit point from the temporal bone (ie, just below the earlobe). Recording electrodes are placed over the facial muscles. The results are compared with the opposite unaffected side and may need to be repeated at different intervals. If Wallerian degeneration has taken place, no response will be detected. This has important implications for prognosis and in deciding if a nerve ought to be surgically explored.

RADIOLOGY

1. *Plain Films.* Plain films and tomography of the temporal bone have almost been rendered obsolete by CT scanning.

2. *Computed Tomographic (CT) Scanning.* High resolution sections 1 to 2 mm thick enable visualization of the detailed bony anatomy of all parts of the ear (Fig 3-7). Soft tissues, such as

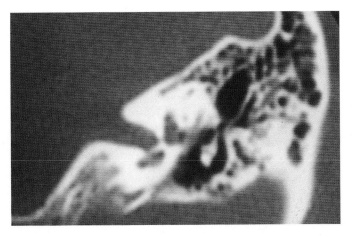

Fig 3-7 CT scan of the ear. This horizontal section shows the normal honeycomb appearance of the mastoid air cells. The heads of the ossicles and the internal auditory canal are also seen.

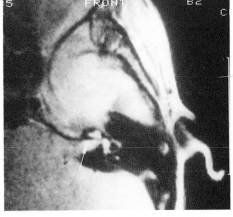

Fig 3-8 MRI. This is a horizontal section. The auditory nerve is well visualized and contains a tiny acoustic neuroma (arrowed). Note the poor visualization of the surrounding bone.

cholesteatoma or acoustic neuroma, can also be clearly seen on these views.

3. *Magnetic Resonance Imaging (MRI).* This investigation has overcome many of the limitations of CT scanning. It is better at imaging soft tissue (such as the auditory or facial nerve) but is poor at defining bone detail. It is excellent at imaging tiny tumors arising from the auditory nerve (acoustic neuromas) or affections of the brain stem (Fig 3-8). Its images can be enhanced by using contrast agents such as gadolinium.

CHAPTER 4

The External Ear

The external ear is a skin-lined structure adapted for sound collection. It comprises the pinna and external ear canal.

AURICULAR HEMATOMA

This typically occurs following blunt injury to the side of the head as may happen in contact sports. The skin of the pinna is tightly bound to the perichondrium of the underlying elastic cartilage. The cartilage depends on perichondrium for its nutrition. A hematoma may detach the perichondrium (Fig 4-1) and cause necrosis of the underlying cartilage, especially if the hematoma becomes infected (perichondritis). Early incision and drainage with strict aseptic technique, usually under anesthesia, is followed by a pressure dressing for 1 week. Broad spectrum antibiotic cover is recommended.

Other types of injury to the pinna include love bites and earring scarring (Figs. 4-2, a and b).

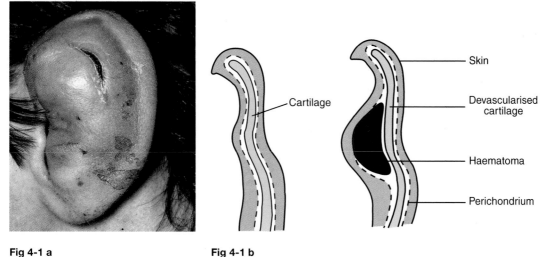

Fig 4-1 a   **Fig 4-1 b**

Fig 4-1 a. Auricular hematoma. **b.** Such a hematoma can devascularize the cartilage.

Fig 4-2 a. This nasty injury to the ear lobe resulted from a love bite. **b.** This deformity resulted from hypertrophic scarring following earring insertion.

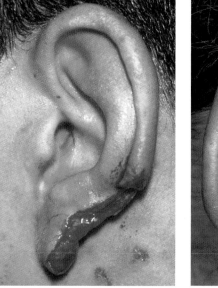

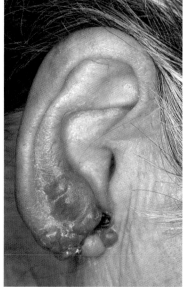

Fig 4-2 a   **Fig 4-2 b**

CAULIFLOWER EAR

If the treatment of perichondritis (Fig 4-3) is neglected (early intravenous antibiotics are essential), the cartilage may shrivel giving rise to this unsightly deformity.

CONGENITAL MALFORMATIONS

These are fully dealt with in the section on pediatric otology (Chapter 8).

IMPACTED WAX

This is a frequent occurrence in general practice, especially in elderly patients (Fig 4-4). The use of cotton swabs to clean the ear usually causes accumulation of wax deep in the meatus, often impacting it against the eardrum. The hearing loss is usually slight, except when the meatus is totally obstructed.

When the wax is hard, soften it by using warm olive oil drops or sodium bicarbonate ear drops for 2 to 3 weeks. Wax removal is rarely an emergency and it is often kinder and safer to do it in stages. Proprietory preparations (cerumolytics) can also be used but they sometimes irritate the skin of the external ear. If wax remains after this therapy, the ear can usually be syringed successfully.

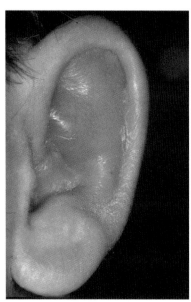

Fig 4-3 Perichondritis. The ear felt hot and was painful. Note the diffuse erythema and swelling. Systemic antibiotics prevented cartilage destruction.

Syringing

Injury to the ear is frequent with this technique, usually because insufficient care is taken in its execution (Figs 4-5 and 4-6). Seat

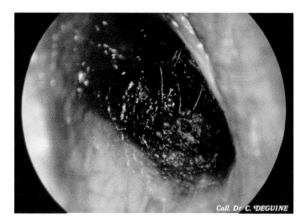

Fig 4-4 Impacted wax. If wax is very hard, it is best softened with olive oil drops over a week or so prior to syringing.

the patient or have him lie on a couch and describe the procedure. *Ask if there is any history of perforation of the eardrum (if there is, syringing is best avoided).*

Check the temperature of the water with a thermometer—it should be warmed precisely to body temperature to avoid caloric stimulation of the labyrinth. Check the syringe—the tip should be blunt and securely attached to the barrel of the syringe. As few patients appreciate being drenched, a protective towel around the neck is desirable.

Steady the patient's head. Gently retract the pinna upward and backward. Syringing must always be done under direct vision. Position the syringe adjacent to the ear canal and inject the water with firm, even pressure. *Direct the flow of water to the back wall of the meatus.* This protects the eardrum from the full force of the stream of water. It also allows the water to get behind the mass of wax and will enable it to be dislodged and flushed outward. After the procedure, dry mop the ear canal with a wisp of cotton wool.

Electrically operated syringes are extremely convenient and the same precautions apply to their use.

> **Key Point:**
> Syringing is contraindicated following recent injury or ear surgery and in patients with a history of perforation of the eardrum.

OTITIS EXTERNA

This is one of the most common affections of the ear. It can be very troublesome to treat if some basic rules are not followed. Otitis externa can be reactive (ie, due to contact allergy) or infective (bacterial, viral, fungal).

Symptoms

The cardinal symptom is *irritation*. It can be intense and often affects both ears simultaneously. Ask about a history of eczema or contact allergy to chemicals, shampoos, or cosmetics. Certain occupations, such as telephone operators who require inserts in their ears, are often affected. Pain occurs only when secondary bacterial infection sets in and hearing loss, if present, is usually mild. Discharge is scanty (there are no mucous secreting glands in the external ear).

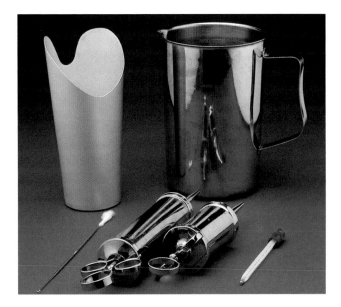

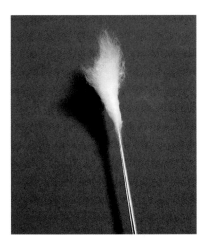

Fig 4-6 Water left behind after ear syringing can be very uncomfortable. Dry mopping the ear canal is recommended.

Fig 4-5 Instruments for ear syringing. A jug for warm water, syringe, thermometer, cotton tip applicator, different sized tips for the syringe, and a receptacle to collect the water.

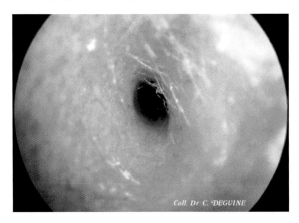

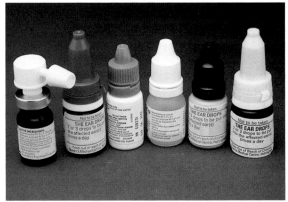

Fig 4-7 An edematous ear canal typical of otitis externa. A microscope is usually required to suction clean such an ear and to insert a dressing with safety.

Fig 4-8 Ear drops come in all shapes and sizes. Remember that ear drops will only work if the ear canal has been properly cleaned.

Treatment

The first consideration is *aural toilet*. Until this is satisfactory, all treatments are doomed to failure. Gentle dry mopping with a wisp of wool on a wool carrier is best—be extremely gentle as the external ear is exquisitely tender. Syringing is best avoided in an acutely inflamed canal. If the ear canal cannot be cleaned or is very narrowed by swelling (Fig 4-7), specialist help may be needed to clean the ear with suction using a microscope.

Once clean, conventional wisdom dictates that a combination of *steroids and antibiotic drops* (Fig 4-8) be given to settle the ear for a week or so. Bear in mind that some patients may be allergic to these drops (Fig 4-9). Prolonged use of antibiotics can give rise to super-infection with yeasts (Figs 4-10 and 4-11) and should be avoided.

Commercially available otowicks (Fig 4-12) that when dry are sufficiently stiff to place in a narrowed canal and that soften and swell when moistened with ear drops, are very helpful.

Advise the patient to keep the ear canal dry as water aggravates otitis externa. Cotton wool smeared with vaseline is an excellent means of achieving this.

Finally, the patient must be persuaded to stop scratching the ear canal with matchsticks, cotton swabs, or fingernails (Fig 4-13). The rule is: *nothing smaller than the elbow in the external ear!*

Some hints on the management of the refractory cases of otitis externa are outlined in Table 4-1.

Key Points:

1. Profuse discharge implies middle ear disease—not otitis externa.

2. Persistent unilateral "otitis externa" equals otitis media until proven otherwise.

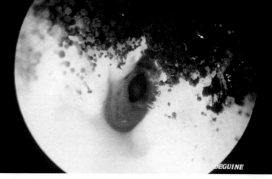

Fig 4-9 Hypersensitivity reaction to ear drops. The pinna is edematous and there is blister formation.

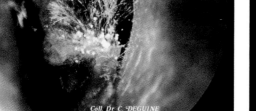

Fig 4-10 Fungal otitis externa. Note the fluffy appearance given by the hyphae. This may follow prolonged treatment with antibacterial ear drops.

Fig 4-11 The striking appearance of clumps of *Aspergillus niger* in the ear canal. Once seen, never forgotten!

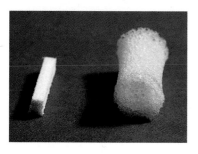

Fig 4-12

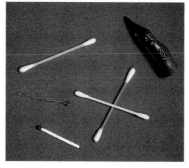

Fig 4-13

Fig 4-12 An otowick. Prior to insertion, it is firm and narrow (left). When drops are applied (left) it softens and expands (right). These are easy to insert even in narrow ear canals (see Fig 4-7).

Fig 4-13 Instruments of torture for the ear canal! Finger nails, cotton swabs, hair clips, and matchsticks are frequently used to scratch the ear canal and cause secondary infection.

Table 4-1. The Stubborn Otitis Externa

Problem	Comment
Aural toilet	If the ear canal is not clean, do not waste time and money changing to yet another brand of ear drops. Either clean the ear or refer to ENT for microsuction.
Fungal infection	Follows prolonged treatment with antibacterial ear drops. Clean the ear and treat with nystatin powder or clotrimazole drops. Fungal otitis externa is often indistinguishable from bacterial otitis externa except for *Aspergillus niger* (see Fig 4-11) whose hyphae form striking black clusters on the canal wall.
Sensitivity to ear drops	Remember that a patient may develop an allergy to ear drops (see Fig 4-9). This can be dramatic and very painful. Always advise patients about this when drops are prescribed.
Hearing aids	The earmold of a hearing aid can alter the humidity of the external ear and predispose to otitis externa. The use of a hearing aid in the acutely inflamed ear is best discouraged. Fit the hearing aid in the other ear where possible and allow the inflammation to subside. A hole can be made in the earmold to allow ventilation of the ear canal in troublesome cases. Allergy to the earmold material should be investigated.
Middle ear disease	Otitis externa can be secondary to middle ear disease. Suspect in unilateral cases and those with profuse discharge.
Microbiology	Should be obtained in difficult cases. Ask for culture for fungi and tuberculosis

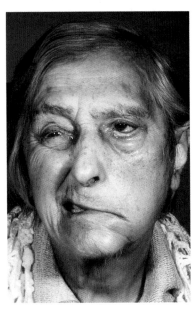

Fig 4-14 Necrotizing "malignant" otitis externa. This elderly diabetic developed otitis externa and facial paralysis. Despite intensive medical and surgical treatment, she succumbed to the disease.

NECROTIZING ("MALIGNANT") OTITIS EXTERNA

This destructive inflammatory process affects immune compromised patients, especially elderly diabetics (Fig 4-14) or other immunocompromised patients (eg, AIDS). The term "malignant" is unfortunate but was applied to this condition to denote its high mortality. It starts as a stubborn otitis externa that gradually causes an osteomyelitis of the skull base. Pain is often severe. Several cranial nerves may be paralyzed, especially the facial nerve and cranial nerves IX to XII. The offending organisms are *Pseudomonas aeruginosa* and anaerobes.

Investigations

Swabs for culture (remember the anaerobes), CT scan or MRI, technetium scan.

Treatment

Intensive local therapy with systemic antibiotics against *Pseudomonas* (ciprofloxacin or ceftazidime being especially effective) and anaerobes is the mainstay of treatment

FURUNCLE OF THE EXTERNAL EAR

This is an infection of a hair follicle—rather like a boil, in the outer third of the ear canal (Fig 4-15). It is excruciatingly painful.

Treatment

Be extremely gentle. Local cleaning of the swollen ear with otowicks (see Fig 4-12) and use of intensive systemic antibiotic therapy against staphylococci are recommended.

FOREIGN BODIES

Foreign bodies often find their way into the ear canal (Fig 4-16, a and b) and can be very difficult to remove. What may at first

> **Key Point:**
> Beware of otitis externa in diabetic and immunocompromised patients.

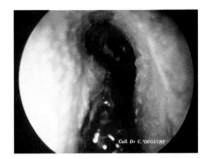

Fig 4-15 Furuncle of the external ear. This infection in a hair follicle of the external ear is excruciatingly painful and the canal is exquisitely tender. In this patient, an abscess has ruptured into the meatus.

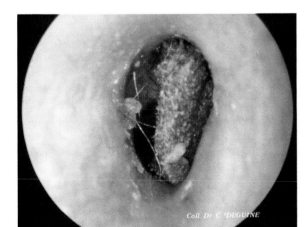

Fig 4-16 a

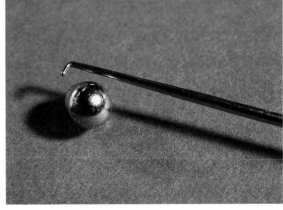

Fig 4-16 b

Fig 4-16 Foreign body deep in the ear canal. **a.** These are best removed by an ENT surgeon. **b.** Beads can be especially difficult to remove and great skill is needed if employing a wax hook to remove them.

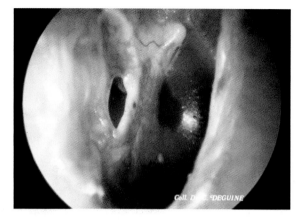

Fig 4-17 Traumatic perforation of the eardrum due to a cotton swab.

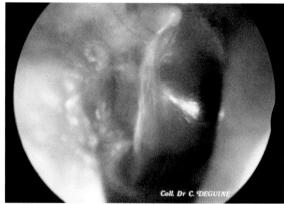

Fig 4-18 The same ear as in Fig 4-17. With masterly inactivity the perforation healed spontaneously in a matter of weeks.

sight seem a trivial technical challenge can soon end up as an inelegant fiasco. The danger is of pushing the object (beads are the worst!) farther into the ear canal causing damage to the eardrum and middle ear. This can easily happen with a fractious child. Vegetable matter can swell and may impact during syringing.

Wax hooks are useful in experienced hands if they can be introduced distal to the foreign body. Foreign bodies that are not readily amenable to removal need referral to an ENT department.

EAR CANAL TRAUMA

This is usually caused by the insertion of cotton swabs and hair clips in the ear (see also Skull Base Trauma, p50). The result is a laceration of the canal and bleeding. It may not be possible to see the ear drum to exclude injury to the middle or inner ear. The treatment is usually one of masterly inactivity (Figs 4-17 and 4-18). The blood clot is best left undisturbed as it acts as a wound dressing. Further evaluation should be carried out after a few weeks.

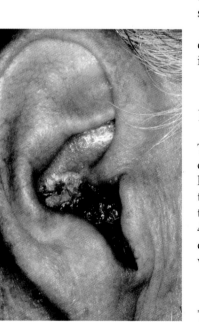

Fig 4-19 This squamous carcinoma of the pinna had raised everted edges. A more common site is on the outer surface of the pinna, especially in those exposed to sunlight.

TUMORS

Pinna

The commonest tumor is a *squamous cell carcinoma* (Fig 4-19) which has an ulcerated appearance with raised everted edges.

Excessive exposure to sunlight is a predisposing factor. This gives rise to solar keratoses which are premalignant. These lesions require early ENT assessment as the prognosis is excellent when the disease is localized. Metastases usually go to the neck. *Basal cell carcinomas* (rodent ulcers) may also affect the pinna. They have a "punched out" appearance. Local invasion rather than distant metastasis is the rule.

Ear Canal

These are uncommon. Benign tumors typically arise from the ceruminous glands. Osteomas (Fig 4-20) may arise from frequent swimming in cold water and need no treatment unless they obstruct the canal.

Malignant primary growths are rare and are usually squamous cell carcinomas. Sometimes the ear canal may be invaded by tumors in adjacent structures, usually the parotid. Deep pain, sometimes accompanied by bloody discharge or facial paralysis, is the hallmark of malignancy (Fig 4-21). Resectable malignant tumors are treated primarily by surgery with or without the addition of radiation therapy.

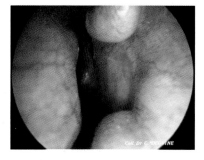

Fig 4-20 Osteomas of the ear canal. These occur in swimmers. They do not require treatment unless they block the ear canal.

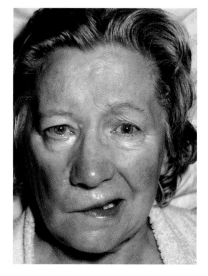

Fig 4-21 Squamous cell carcinoma of the ear canal. The patient was treated for many months for "otitis externa." The pain was intense and facial paralysis set in. The patient's facies conveys her distress.

CHAPTER 5

The Middle Ear

The middle ear contains the chain of bones necessary for sound conduction (Fig 5-1). It is bounded laterally by the tympanic membrane, medially by the inner ear, and anteriorly by the eustachian tube. The roof is a wafer thin bone, which separates the middle ear from the middle fossa dura. Behind, the middle ear communicates with the mastoid air cell system, which is closely related to the posterior cranial fossa. Entwined in this tiny space is the facial nerve, which pursues a tortuous course through the middle ear.

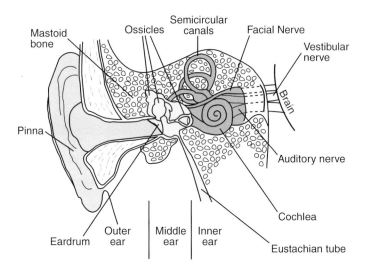

Fig 5-1 The middle ear and its immediate relationships. Note that only a thin layer of bone (the tegmen tympani) separates the middle ear from the middle cranial fossa.

The following conditions are described in the chapter on pediatric otology:

Acute otitis media (see p62)

Recurrent otitis media (see p63)

Acute mastoiditis and masked mastoiditis (see p64)

Otitis media with effusion (chronic serous otitis media, "glue" ear) (see p65)

MIDDLE EAR EFFUSIONS IN ADULTS

Typically these follow upper respiratory tract infection or barotrauma. Patients with nasal obstruction (polyps, allergic, or vasomotor rhinitis) may also develop fluid in their middle ears. Unilateral effusion in an adult should always be viewed with suspicion. A nasopharyngeal tumor may invade the muscles surrounding the eustachian tube and thus prevent its opening. This applies especially to southern Chinese patients in whom this tumor is endemic.

> **Key Point:**
> Unilateral serous effusion in an adult is due to nasopharyngeal tumor until proven otherwise.

CHRONIC SUPPURATIVE OTITIS MEDIA

There are two varieties: "safe" and "unsafe." The latter is more important as it refers to a destructive process. It is usually due to cholesteatoma. The safe variety implies a simple chronic discharge from the ear without the destructive sequelae typical of cholesteatoma.

CHRONIC SUPPURATIVE OTITIS MEDIA WITH CHOLESTEATOMA

Cholesteatoma

This is the term given to keratinizing squamous epithelium in the middle ear. The cause is unknown. It is possible that persistent negative pressure in the middle ear causes the tympanic membrane to be sucked inward, resulting in retraction pocket formation (Figs 5-2 and 5-3). The skin desquamates causing expansion of these pockets that invariably become infected. These "skin bags" are locally destructive to all the structures in the temporal bone.

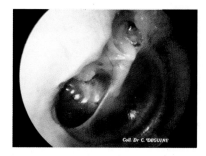

Fig 5-2 Retraction pockets. These form when the tympanic membrane gets "sucked into" the middle ear. Gradually the pocket deepens and fills with desquamating epithelium. Compare with Fig 5-3.

Symptoms

Smelly discharge from an ear is the hallmark of this condition. Invariably, the discharge is accompanied by hearing loss. If the inner ear is eroded, the patient may become vertiginous or lose hearing completely. Pressure on the facial nerve can cause paralysis of the face.

Spread of infection outside the ear may result in intracranial suppuration (see p40), usually affecting the temporal lobe.

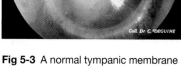

Fig 5-3 A normal tympanic membrane for comparison.

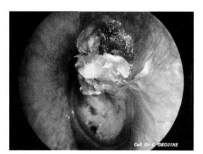

Fig 5-4 An attic crust. Beneath such a crust usually lurks a cholesteatoma.

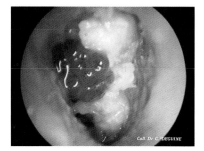

Fig 5-5 Cholesteatoma. It was originally described as a "pearly tumor" due to its whitish, glistening appearance. Note the granulation tissue that often accompanies cholesteatoma.

Key Points:

1. Smelly discharge from the ear strongly suggests cholesteatoma.

2. Suppurative ear disease is still the commonest cause of temporal lobe abscess.

3. A discharging mastoid cavity is no safer than a discharging ear. These patients should be considered for revision surgery.

4. The main risks of mastoid surgery are sensorineural hearing loss, vertigo, and facial paralysis.

Examination

Otoscopy reveals debris in the ear canal. Look with care at the attic area (the uppermost part of the eardrum) in these cases. Here you will see either a crust (Fig 5-4) or a perforation full of whitish debris (Fig 5-5). Tuning forks usually indicate a conductive hearing loss. Culture from the discharge usually grows *Pseudomas aeruginosa* and anaerobes.

Investigations

Examination under the microscope, audiometry, microbiology, and CT scans are occasionally indicated.

Treatment

Once the diagnosis is made (and it is easy to do so) it is pointless to persist with ear drops and antibiotics. Surgical treatment, usually a mastoid exploration, is necessary to treat the condition.

The main priority for the surgeon is to remove the diseased area and render the patient safe from the threat of continued suppuration. Following mastoid surgery the ear should be dry and trouble free. Regular follow up will be needed for life as cholesteatomas can recur. To improve hearing, reconstruction of the ossicular chain (ossiculoplasty) may be feasible at a later stage. Provided the ear is dry following surgery, the patient also has the option of wearing a hearing aid. A patient with a persistently discharging ear following previous surgery should be offered a revision procedure.

CHRONIC SUPPURATIVE OTITIS MEDIA— WITHOUT CHOLESTEATOMA

In this condition, the problem is caused by perforation of the pars tensa (Fig 5-6). External and nasopharyngeal infection can easily gain access to the middle ear, irritating the mucosa and causing increased mucous production (Figs 5-7 and 5-8)—it is rather like chronic bronchitis in the ear! Unlike cholesteatoma, the discharge is not offensive but is just as copious. Typically, there is hearing impairment.

Examination

Otoscopy reveals a perforation in the pars tensa. Tuning fork testing will suggest conductive hearing impairment.

Investigations

Audiogram, microsuction, culture, and sensitivity (occasionally).

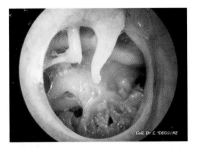

Fig 5-6 A large pars tensa perforation (right ear). The malleus handle, long process of incus, stapedius muscle, round window niche, and promontory can be seen.

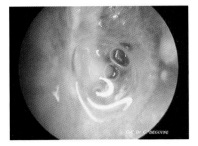

Fig 5-7 Chronic suppurative otitis media—"safe." During an exacerbation mucoid discharge fills the ear canal.

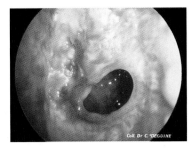

Fig 5-8 Chronic suppurative otitis media—"safe." The same ear as in Fig 5-7 following microsuction. A central perforation through which can be seen an angry-looking, hyperemic middle ear mucosa.

Treatment

Medical management (debridement, antibiotic/steroid drops, keeping the ear dry) can often resolve matters to the patient's satisfaction. Ear drops that contain ototoxic compounds are best avoided in the presence of a perforation. A hearing aid, which works well for conductive losses, may need to be considered. If medical therapy fails or if the patient is keen on surgery (for instance, to allow swimming or for occupational reasons) then the defect can be grafted (myringoplasty). With any operation on the ear there is a small risk of sensorineural hearing loss and there is the possibility of graft failure.

> **Key Point:**
> Perforations of the pars tensa lend themselves well to surgical repair.

TYMPANOSCLEROSIS

This term is applied to "chalk patches" in the tympanic membrane or middle ear (Fig 5-9). A horseshoe-shaped ring of tympanosclerosis often follows grommet insertion. The process starts as hyalin degeneration followed by calcification. When tympanosclerosis is confined to the tympanic membrane it is rarely associated with hearing loss.

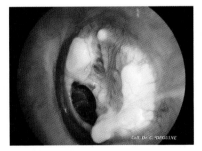

Fig 5-9 Tympanosclerosis ("chalk patches"). Degenerative changes can result in plaques of calcification in the tympanic membrane or middle ear.

TUBERCULOUS OTITIS MEDIA

An important cause of suppuration in developing countries, this diagnosis should be considered in ears that fail to respond to standard therapy, especially in patients from third world countries with multiple perforations of the eardrum. A swab for appropriate culture studies coupled with a chest X ray will usually confirm the diagnosis.

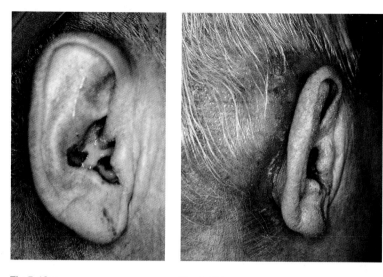

Fig 5-10 a   **Fig 5-10 b**

Fig 5-10 a. and b. Intracranial complication of ear disease. This patient presented to casualty with headache, a swelling above the ear, and profuse smelly discharge.

INTRACRANIAL COMPLICATIONS OF EAR INFECTION

The most serious complication of acute or chronic suppuration in an ear is intracranial sepsis (Figs 5-10, a and b, and 5-11). The most important warning signs are headache and deep pain in the ear (Table 5-1). Uncomplicated chronic ear disease is not painful. Patients with such a history should be sent for urgent ENT assessment.

Management

Patients should be managed in consultation with a neurosurgeon. A CT scan of the brain is essential. Lumbar puncture should not be performed in patients with raised intracranial pressure. A

Table 5-1. Intracranial Suppuration From Ear Disease

Diagnosis	Clinical Features
Meningitis	Neck stiffness, photophobia, positive Kernig's sign, etc.
Lateral sinus thrombosis	Headache, rigors, spiking temperature, papilloedema, positive blood culture
Temporal lobe abscess	Headaches, drowsiness, visual field defects, dysphasia, etc.
Cerebellar abscess	Headaches, ataxia, cerebellar signs, neck stiffness, etc.

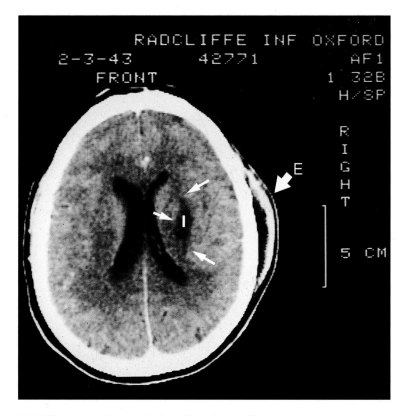

Fig 5-11 Intracranial complication of ear disease. The same patient as in Fig 5-10. CT scan. There is an abscess in the temporal lobe (I) as well as a large collection of pus extracranially (E). The source of infection was cholesteatoma.

brain abscess will need repeated aspiration and intensive antibiotic therapy. The definitive treatment of the underlying ear disease is best carried out when the patient's condition has stabilized.

OTOSCLEROSIS

This condition affects the dense otic capsule bone that houses the inner ear. New spongy bone is formed in the region of the stapes footplate (Fig 5-12). This inhibits the mobility of the footplate resulting in conductive hearing loss. The condition is usually bilateral and symmetrical. It is inherited as a Mendelian autosomal dominant trait with incomplete penetrance. About half the patients have a positive family history. Its onset is typically in the second or third decades with a slightly higher incidence in females. The condition tends to be precipitated or promoted by pregnancy.

Key Points:

1. The complaint of earache or headache in a patient with chronic ear disease should suggest the possibility of intracranial complication.

2. A normal CT scan does not exclude intracranial suppuration.

3. Early neurosurgical consultation should be obtained for patients with suspected or established intracranial disease.

4. Suspect disease in the ear (or nose) in a patient with recurrent attacks of bacterial meningitis.

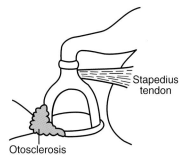

Stapedius tendon

Otosclerosis

Fig 5-12 Otosclerosis. New spongy bone is laid down in the region of the stapes footplate. This causes fixation of the stapes and conductive hearing loss. The eardrum is normal.

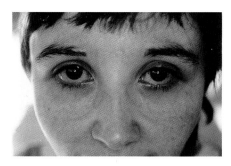

Fig 5-13 Van der Hoeve's syndrome. This describes the association between osteogenesis imperfecta, blue sclerae, and otosclerosis.

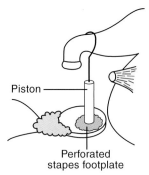

Piston

Perforated stapes footplate

Fig 5-14 Stapedectomy. The arch of the stapes is removed and is replaced by a piston, thus restoring the mobility of the ossicular chain.

Key Point:

A normal eardrum in a patient with conductive hearing loss suggests otosclerosis.

The association of osteogenesis imperfecta (brittle bone disease), blue sclerae, and otosclerosis is called Van der Hoeve's syndrome (Fig 5-13).

Diagnosis

The presence of a *normal eardrum* in a patient with *conductive hearing loss* usually implies otosclerosis.

Treatment

Options for treatment are outlined in Table 5-2.

Table 5-2. Treatment Options in Otosclerosis

No treatment	This is often the best option, especially when the hearing loss is slight or unilateral.
Hearing aid	Hearing aids work very effectively in conductive losses, especially when inner ear function is normal. This is because all that is required is amplification. Patients with otosclerosis should be encouraged to try a hearing aid prior to embarking on surgery.
Stapedectomy	This operation involves removing the stapes and replacing it with a piston (Fig 5-14). The operation results in a dramatic and prolonged hearing gain. It carries a small but definite risk of sensorineural hearing loss.

CHAPTER 6

The Inner Ear

Inner ear disorders manifest themselves with sensorineural hearing loss, tinnitus, vertigo, or facial paralysis.

ACOUSTIC NEUROMA

These are benign tumors which arise from the auditory nerve. The tumors arise in the internal auditory canal (Fig 6-1). Later, they expand causing cranial nerve palsies, brain stem compression, and raised intracranial pressure. Patients with neurofibromatosis type 2 may have bilateral tumors, and should be differentiated from neurofibromatosis type 1 (von Recklinghausen's disease), who are

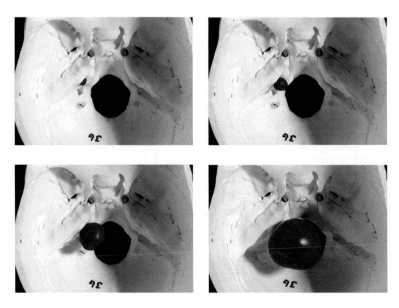

Fig 6-1 The growth of acoustic neuromas. These tumors arise in the internal auditory canal (intracanalicular) (upper left). Typical 1 cm (lower left), 2 cm (upper right), and 4 cm tumor (lower right) are shown. Note how these tumors can impinge on the brain stem as they enlarge.

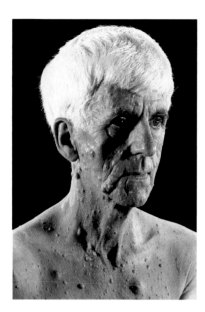

Fig 6-2 Neurofibromatosis type 1 (von Recklinghausen's disease). Note the typical cutaneous neurofibromata. These patients do not typically develop acoustic neuromas.

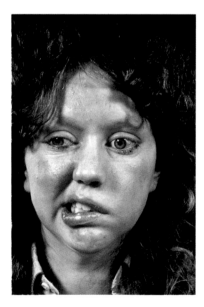

Fig 6-3 Neurofibromatosis type 2. This 22 year old girl had *bilateral* acoustic tumors. The tumor on the left side was removed leaving her with a facial paralysis and a "dead" ear. The acoustic neuroma in the right ear will be allowed to remain as long as her hearing lasts, provided her neurological condition remains stable.

typically spared the development of intracranial neuromas (Figs 6-2 and 6-3).

The earliest symptom is *unilateral hearing loss or tinnitus.* Sometimes the hearing loss can be of sudden onset. Vertigo is uncommon. Patients with large tumors experience headaches, visual disturbance, and ataxia.

Early diagnosis is crucial as the mortality and morbidity from surgery is directly related to tumor size. For instance, small tumors can be removed with preservation of the facial nerve (and sometimes hearing). The removal of large tumors can compromise the blood supply to the brain stem, and preservation of the facial nerve is rarely possible. The complications are thus formidable.

Investigations

Pure tone audiometry will usually confirm unilateral or asymmetrical sensorineural hearing loss. Electric response audiometry (Fig 6-4) is a valuable screening tool to differentiate cochlear deafness from deafness due to tumors on the auditory nerve (retrocochlear disease). A caloric test will reveal an absent or depressed response. Magnetic resonance imaging (Fig 6-5) gives the definitive diagnosis.

Treatment

1. Three management strategies exist. Interval scanning where the patient elects to be followed with serial MRI scans until the tumor exhibits significant enlargement.

2. Stereotactically guided radiation treatment (sometimes referred to as the gamma knife). This treatment avoids surgery,

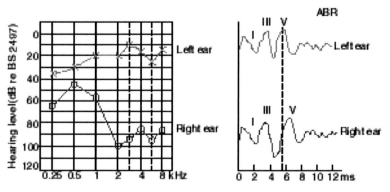

Fig 6-4 Pure tone audiogram and auditory brainstem responses in a patient with a right sided acoustic neuroma. The hearing is normal in the left ear as is the I–V latency (broken vertical line represents upper limit of normal). On the right side, there is high frequency hearing loss and the I–V latency is prolonged. (*Note*: Wave I—distal cochlear nerve, Wave III—cochlear nuclei, and Wave V–tracts and nuclei lateral lemniscus).

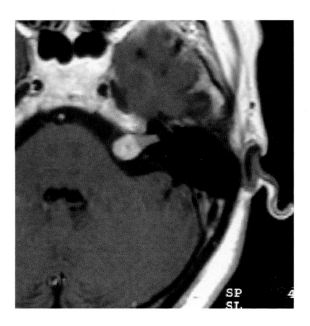

Fig 6-5 This MRI scan clearly demonstrates this acoustic neuroma in a patient who presented with unilateral hearing loss.

but the radiation may have long-term effects on adjacent tissue. There is no evidence radiation treatment works better than interval scanning.

3. Surgical removal. This is undertaken microsurgically by a neurosurgeon and an otologist working as a team. Physiological monitoring of the facial and auditory nerves during surgery has greatly improved the functional outcome (Fig 6-6). The

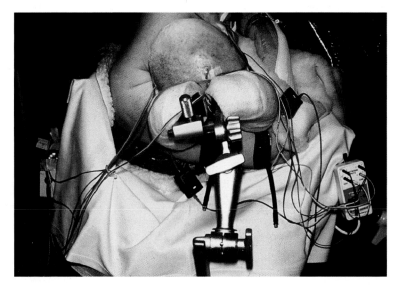

Fig 6-6
Neuromonitoring. During surgery for acoustic tumors, use is made of physiological monitoring to monitor hearing and facial nerve function.

disadvantages of surgery are those inherent in any intracranial procedure, with specific risks to hearing and the facial nerves.

PRESBYACUSIS

This is the term applied to hearing loss due to aging. It is usually bilateral and symmetrical (Fig 6-7). The age of onset is variable.

Audiometry often reveals a high-frequency loss. The high frequencies are crucial for speech intelligibility. Consonants (/d/, /n/, /t/, /l/, /s/), which act as the "stop gaps" in speech are generally in the high frequency range (Fig 6-8). Vowels tend to be low frequency and are less important for understanding speech (Table 6-1).

Many patients with presbyacusis become unduly sensitive to certain sounds. This is because the cochlea loses its ability to accommodate its normally vast intensity range (over 1 million to one!) resulting in abnormal growth of loudness (called *recruitment*). This explains why shouting at a patient with high-frequency sensorineural loss often adds nothing to what they understand and may make matters worse.

Thus, many of these patients complain that while they know people are speaking they cannot understand what is being said. They often say that words merge one into the other or that the speech is "muffled." They function well on a one-to-one basis but have great difficulty with group conversation and when there is background noise.

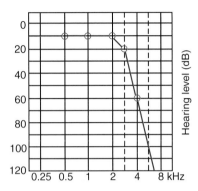

Fig 6-7 Presbyacusis. The typical audiogram shows high frequency bilateral symmetrical sensorineural hearing loss.

Management

Many patients are concerned that they may lose their hearing completely and reassurance on this front is important. Emphasizing their good low and mid-frequency hearing is good for morale. It is also very useful to explain to patients and their relatives the communication difficulties caused by high-frequency hearing loss as this makes all parties more tolerant. Many, however, will need a properly fitted hearing aid which for most patients will offer substantial hearing improvement (see Chapter 9).

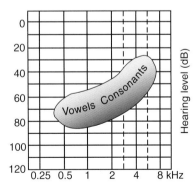

Fig 6-8 The representation of vowels and consonants on a pure tone audiogram. Consonants are more important for understanding speech. Many patients with high-frequency loss can hear the spoken voice but cannot make out what is being said.

Table 6-1. The Relative Importance of Vowels and Consonants

By removing consonants (high frequency) from the sentence, no intelligible message remains. Removing vowels (low frequency) has much less effect.

Example : *"The cat sat on the bag."*

Without consonants	*e a a o e a*
Without vowels	*Th c t s t n th b g*

SUDDEN SENSORINEURAL HEARING LOSS

This is a medical emergency and patients should have the benefit of urgent ENT assessment. The hearing loss may be associated with a constitutional upset, often attributed to viral illness. The more severe cases tend to be accompanied by vertigo.

Management—Early

Bed rest is helpful initially along with vasodilators such as cinnarizine or betahistine. Carbogen gas (a mixture of 5% CO_2 and 95% O_2) is advocated by some to improve oxygen delivery to the damaged cochlea. *Steroids* may be given in a reducing dose over 5 days, provided there are no medical contraindications.

Management—Late

It is essential to exclude an acoustic neuroma or other disease (eg, syphilitic disease) in the auditory system.

Prognosis

This needs to be guarded. In general, low-frequency losses recover better than high frequency deficits and severe vertigo is an unfavorable prognostic factor. Recovery usually takes place within 2 to 4 weeks but there are some late recoveries.

MÉNIÈRE'S DISEASE

This clinical condition, which tends to be overdiagnosed, is characterized by intermittent attacks of vertigo, fluctuant hearing loss, and tinnitus. Very often, there is a sensation of pressure in the affected ear, which may warn the patient of an impending attack. The hearing loss affects the low frequencies initially and is sensorineural in type. Later, the other frequencies may be affected. Occasionally, the condition may be bilateral. The vertigo usually lasts between 10 minutes and 8 hours and is often accompanied by nausea and vomiting. The condition most commonly affects adults (women more than men) between the ages of 35 and 55.

The cause of this condition is unknown but there is no shortage of ideas. Among the possible mechanisms are immunological, vascular, endocrine, heredity, and psychological factors.

Pathology

Excessive accumulation of endolymphatic fluid (hydrops) is the most commonly observed finding. The distension may result in rupture of the inner ear membranes and mixing of endolymph

---

Key Point:

Aging affects both sides of the body! It does not typically cause unilateral hearing loss (cf. acoustic neuroma).

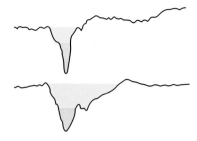

Fig 6-9 A normal electrocochleogram (above). Note the changes typical of an excess of fluid in the endolymph compartment (endolymphatic hydrops), as occurs in Ménière's disease (below).

(which is rich in potassium) and perilymph (which is low in potassium). This is the basis for the abrupt cochleovestibular failure that characterizes this condition.

Investigations

Pure tone audiometry. Evoked response audiometry is useful in excluding a retrocochlear cause (ie, an acoustic neuroma) and electrocochleography (Fig 6-9) may sometimes be diagnostic. Serological testing to exclude syphilitic ear disease should be performed. CT scanning and MRI may be necessary to exclude acoustic neuroma.

Treatment

The natural history of Ménière's disease is decidedly toward spontaneous resolution. Reassurance is therefore extremely important.

Medical: Acute Phase

Bed rest, vestibular sedatives (diazepam is best), antiemetics (phenothiazines).

Prophylaxis

This is an area of some controversy. Betahistine has been shown to supress histamine receptors in the vestibular nuclei and may thus help control troublesome dysequilibrium; it may also improve the cochlear microcirculation. Salt restriction also has its advocates.

Surgery

This is reserved for medical failures and thus has only a limited place in the treatment of Ménière's disease. Hearing conservation procedures (decompression of the endolymphatic sac, division of the vestibular nerve) are preferred to procedures that destroy inner ear function (total labyrinthectomy).

ACUTE VESTIBULAR FAILURE (VESTIBULAR NEURONITIS)

In this condition, there is a sudden, severe onset of incapacitating vertigo in a previously healthy patient. The patients are usually aged between 20 to 40. An important feature is the absence of hearing loss or tinnitus. The duration of the acute attack varies between 2 and 5 days, with mild dysequilibrium persisting over

---

Key Points:

1. The diagnosis of Ménière's disease requires a triad of symptoms (fluctuant hearing loss, tinnitus and vertigo). All that spins is not Ménière's disease!

2. Spontaneous resolution occurs in over 70% of patients with Ménière's disease.

3. Consider the diagnosis of acoustic neuroma in all patients with unilateral inner ear symptoms.

several weeks (Table 6-2). Examination confirms the presence of spontaneous nystagmus. Treatment is symptomatic (vestibular sedatives, especially diazepam in the initial stage). The cause is unknown but is often considered to be viral and the prognosis is excellent.

BENIGN POSITIONAL VERTIGO (BPV)

This condition is characterized by intermittent attacks of vertigo on adopting a sudden change in posture, ie, on lying down, stooping, etc. It often follows head injury. The attacks last a few seconds and are not associated with any auditory symptoms (Table 6-2). Positional testing (Figs 6-10 and 6-11) is pathogno-monic of this condition. Treatment is helped by targeted physical rehabilitation exercises and the prognosis is excellent although recovery may take up to 2 years.

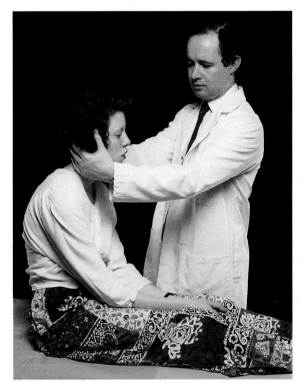

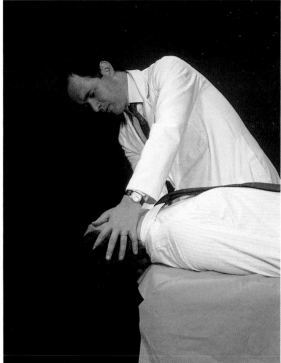

Fig 6-10 Positional testing. The starting position of the patient on the couch must be such as to allow the head to be dropped below the end of the bed when the patient is thrust into a horizontal position (see Fig 6-11).

Fig 6-11 Positional testing. Note that the head is below the level of the couch and rotated to one side. The patient's eyes should be open to observe nystagmus. With the affected ear lowermost, a rotatory nystagmus is produced after a latent period of a second or so. Repeated testing produces a progressively smaller response (fatigability).

BAROTRAUMA AND PERILYMPH FISTULA

In the inner ear the two fluid chambers are separated by extremely delicate membranes. Sudden pressure changes, such as may occur during flying or diving (or even sneezing or straining), may rupture these membranes causing mixing of the biochemically different fluids in the inner ear. This results in any combination of sensorineural hearing loss, tinnitus, and vertigo (see Table 6-2). The fistula test (p18) may be positive. Many leaks seal spontaneously on bed rest. Closure of the leak is possible surgically and this typically alleviates the vertigo.

TRAUMA TO THE EAR AND SKULL BASE

Fractures of the temporal bone can be either longitudinal (80%) or transverse (20%). This is fortunate as transverse fractures cause more damage to the inner ear and facial nerve.

Examination

There are a number of important physical findings: hematoma over the mastoid bone (Battle's sign) (Fig 6-12); blood in the external ear; laceration along the roof of the external ear; CSF otorrhea or rhinorrhoea (if the drum is intact, the CSF escapes down the eustachian tube) (Figs 6-13 and 6-14); blood behind an intact ear drum (hemotympanum); conductive hearing loss from fluid in the middle ear or disruption of the ossicular chain; sensorineural hearing loss from cochlear fracture or concussion. The timing of onset of a facial paralysis (Figs 6-15 and 6-16) is important to ascertain.

Treatment

General care of a patient with head injury is necessary. Facial paralysis may call for exploration of the facial nerve and microneural repair. Conductive hearing loss may require ossiculoplasty at a

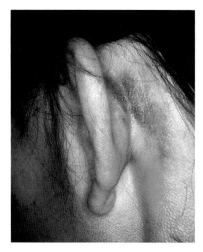

Fig 6-12 Battle's sign. A hematoma over the mastoid is sometimes seen following temporal bone fracture.

Table 6-2. The Differential Diagnosis of Peripheral Vertigo

Diagnosis	Duration of Vertigo	Hearing Loss/Tinnitus
Ménière's disease	10 min–10 hrs	yes
Acute vestibular failure (vestibular neuronitis)	2–5 days	none
Benign positional vertigo	seconds	none
Perilymphatic fistula	months to years	yes
Psychogenic	years	none

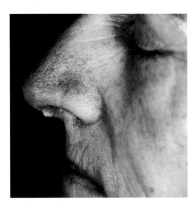

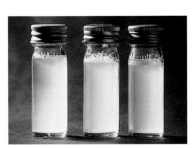

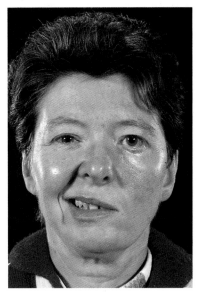

Fig 6-13 CSF rhinorrhoea. This patient was referred because of a long-standing "runny nose." Twelve years previously she had sustained a skull base fracture. Note the drip on the nasal tip. The unilateral rhinorrhea had been attributed mistakenly to sinusitis!

Fig 6-14 CSF rhinorrhea. The same patient as in Fig 6-13. After bending over for half an hour this amount of fluid was produced. The leak was repaired.

Fig 6-15 Fractured temporal bone. This fracture involved the ear, producing a conductive hearing loss and facial paralysis.

Fig 6-16 Fractured temporal bone—CT scan. This fracture line traversed the inner ear causing total sensorineural hearing loss.

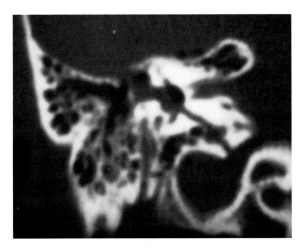

later stage. CSF rhinorrhea will usually settle spontaneously but may need surgical repair. Persistent vertigo or imbalance may point to rupture of either the round or oval windows.

NOISE-INDUCED HEARING LOSS

The inner ear can be damaged by sudden acoustic trauma (eg, blast injury, gunfire, etc) or by prolonged exposure to excessive noise. In acute injury, the sensorineural hearing impairment is greatest at very high frequencies and is often accompanied by

Key Points:

1. Total facial paralysis immediately following head injury suggests major injury to the nerve. Delayed paralysis usually recovers spontaneously.

2. The ear canal should not be syringed in patients with temporal bone fractures.

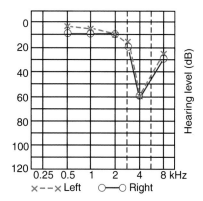

Fig 6-17 Noise-induced hearing loss. The external ear canal acts as a tube that resonates at 4 kHz. Hence the dip at this frequency following noise exposure.

Key Points:

1. To attribute hearing loss to noise requires the patient to have had a genuine history of noise exposure. If the loss is not symmetrical, investigate for acoustic neuroma.

2. Cotton wool plugs may keep dust out of ear canals—they do not protect from noise.

---

tinnitus. With prolonged exposure, as in heavy industry, the hearing loss may be reversible initially. This is due to cochlear fatigue and is called a *temporary threshold shift*. This usually occurs within 2 hours of exposure. With further exposure, a permanent threshold shift occurs. The typical audiogram shows a notch at 4 kHz (Fig 6-17) with gradual involvement of the lower frequencies with continued exposure.

The law requires that workers be protected from noise and strict criteria for permissible levels have been laid down. The damaging effects of noise may be minimized in a number of ways: by reducing the noise output from machines, by wearing ear defenders (cotton wool plugs do not protect from noise!), by keeping to a minimum the duration of exposure to the noise, by offering rest intervals, and by having regular screening audiometry of personnel at risk.

AIDS AND THE EAR

The acquired immune deficiency syndrome (AIDS) can affect the ear. The major manifestations of this disorder are summarized in Table 6-3.

Table 6-3. Acquired Immune Deficiency Syndrome and the Ear

External ear	Kaposi's sarcoma, fungal otitis externa, necrotizing ("malignant") otitis.
Middle ear	Acute and serous otitis media. Mastoiditis. Most common in pediatric AIDS.
Inner ear	Sensorineural hearing loss (neuropathy of the auditory nerve). Iatrogenic (vincristine, antifungal agents). Hearing loss progresses with disease. Exclude neurosyphilis.

OTOTOXICITY

The principal groups of drugs injurious to the inner ear are the aminoglycosides, diuretics (eg, frusemide), salicylates, and chemotherapeutic agents. Some drugs selectively damage the cochlea (neomycin, kanamycin) while others damage the vestibular system (streptomycin). Gentamicin damages both systems.

Tinnitus is usually the first symptom, followed by progressive sensorineural hearing loss and vertigo.

Prevention is crucially important as there is little one can do to reverse the damaging effects of these drugs. Great care must be taken in patients with compromised renal function. Monitoring serum levels during treatment is essential. Serial audiometry is helpful. The use of nonototoxic alternatives (ie, cephalosporins) should always be considered. Ear drops containing ototoxics may carry a risk of damage to the inner ear.

GLOMUS TUMORS

These rare benign tumors arise from nonchromaffin paraganglionic tissue, which has a wide distribution in the head and neck. In the neck, these cells give rise to carotid body tumors (p222). In the temporal bone, 3 types of tumor may arise depending on location: glomus tympanicum (arising in the middle ear), glomus jugulare (arising in the jugular bulb), and glomus vagale (arising near the point of exit of the vagus nerve from the temporal bone).

Symptoms

Tinnitus synchronous with the pulse beat is the classic symptom. Hearing loss (conductive or sensorineural), facial paralysis, and paralysis of cranial nerves IX to XII may occur.

Examination

A pulsatile mass behind the eardrum ("setting sun" sign) (Fig 6-18) is usually apparent. Sometimes an audible bruit over the temporal bone, facial paralysis, or paralysis of cranial nerves IX to XII may be present.

Treatment

Surgery, radiation therapy, or a combination of both.

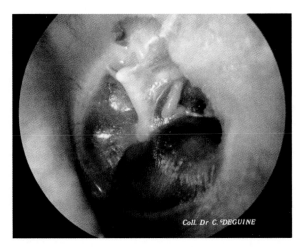

Fig 6-18 Glomus jugulare. These benign tumors arise from the jugular bulb, giving rise to the "setting sun" sign shown here.

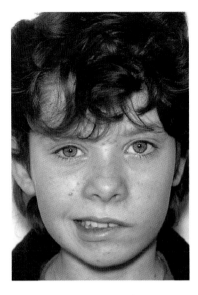

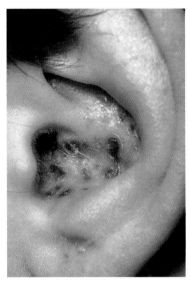

Fig 6-19 Herpes zoster oticus—Ramsay Hunt syndrome. The patient developed earache, followed by a vesicular eruption and facial paralysis (see Fig 7-1).

Fig 6-20 Herpes zoster oticus—Ramsay Hunt syndrome. The characteristic vesicular eruption.

HERPES ZOSTER OTICUS (RAMSAY HUNT SYNDROME)

The herpes zoster virus may attack the spiral or vestibular ganglion in the inner ear or the ganglia of the facial nerve. The first symptom is intense pain in the ear (with little to be found on examination), followed a few days later by a vesicular eruption on the pinna and external ear. Sensorineural deafness, vertigo, and facial paralysis may ensue (Ramsay Hunt syndrome) (Figs 6-19 and 6-20). Early treatment with the antiviral agent acyclovir is said to improve prognosis and reduce the likelihood of postherpetic neuralgia.

TINNITUS

Tinnitus is an hallucination of noises in the head or ears. It is a description of a symptom and not a diagnosis. It may occur on its own or be associated with hearing loss and vertigo. In certain unfortunate patients it can prove to be almost unbearable and drive them to distraction. Some such patients have committed suicide.

Management

These patients need careful neurotological assessment, especially those with unilateral symptoms (bear in mind Ménière's disease, acoustic neuroma, glomus jugulare tumors, intracranial vascular abnormality).

Once underlying disease is excluded, patient counselling is perhaps the most important aspect of management. Most patients can manage tinnitus with their own resources provided they have been given sufficient reassurance. For those with hearing impairment, a hearing aid may be invaluable (by hearing better, the patient is distracted from the underlying tinnitus). If getting to sleep is a problem, using the "snooze" facility on a clock radio may be helpful. In others, nighttime sedation may be required. Self help and support groups are useful and help patients maintain their morale.

Those patients distressed by their tinnitus should be referred to specialist tinnitus clinics for specialist counselling, *Tinnitus maskers* (p77) and tinnitus retraining therapy.

NONORGANIC HEARING LOSS

It is important to recognize nonorganic hearing loss and it often represents a pitfall for the unwary. It is most likely to occur in the pursuit of compensation following head injury or alleged injurious exposure to noise. Other patients may feign total deafness to fulfill some psychological need (adolescent girls most commonly).

Diagnosis depends on awareness and a number of audiological tests have been developed to support clinical suspicions. Electric response audiometry will ultimately confirm the diagnosis.

CHAPTER 7

The Facial Nerve

The cell bodies of the facial nerve lie in the facial nuclei of the brain stem. The nerve leaves the brain stem in the cerebellopontine angle, directing its way towards the internal auditory canal. It then enters the temporal bone and has a complex "Z"-shaped course through it. Its course within bone is the longest of any nerve in the body—about 30 mm. Having left the temporal bone it then enters the parotid gland and fans out to supply the muscles of facial expression.

The cerebellopontine angle, temporal bone, and parotid gland are havens of pathology. Thus it makes sense to consider lower motor neuron facial paralysis under the headings: intracranial, intratemporal, and extratemporal (Table 7-1).

Table 7-1 Causes of Lower Motor Neuron Paralysis

Intracranial	Intratemporal	Extratemporal
Meningioma	Acute and chronic ear disease	Parotid malignancy
Congenital cholesteatoma	Glomus tumors	Facial lacerations
Acoustic neuroma	Herpes zoster	
	Fracture	
	Postsurgery	
	Temporal bone tumor	
	Bell's palsy	

Patients with facial paralysis need careful history taking, ENT, and neurological examination. Always examine the parotid gland—remember it has a deep lobe which may displace a tonsil and can be seen and felt through the mouth. Partial paralysis or bilateral paralysis can easily be overlooked (Figs 7-1–7-7).

Photography of facial movements is an excellent method of recording the degree of paralysis. Audiometry and measurements of stapedial reflexes are necessary in most cases. Electroneuronography (p25) can evaluate the severity of nerve injury and give a guide to progress and prognosis. Magnetic resonance imaging and CT scanning are indicated in selected patients.

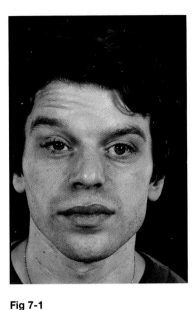

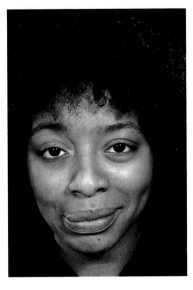

Fig 7-1

Fig 7-2

Fig 7-1 Facial paralyis (left) due to invasion of the nerve by a glomus jugulare tumour.

Fig 7-2 This mild facial paralysis could be easily overlooked. It was due to pathology at the petrous apex.

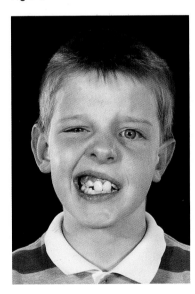

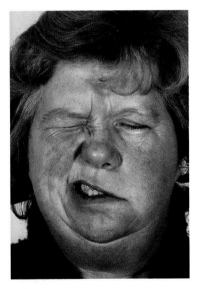

Fig 7-3

Fig 7-4

Fig 7-3 Facial paralysis in a young boy following a road traffic accident.

Fig 7-4 This idiopathic (Bell's palsy) facial paralysis fully recovered over a 2-month period.

BELL'S PALSY

The diagnosis of Bell's palsy should only be applied when no specific cause has been found for a facial paralysis after thorough investigation (Figs 7-5–7-7). Typically the paralysis is of sudden onset and is complete within 24 hours. Signs of recovery begin to appear within 2 months of the onset. Steroids are probably useful if given early in the course of the condition.

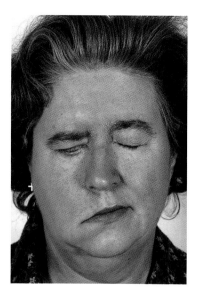

Fig 7-5 This facial paralysis was due to involvement of the nerve by a malignant parotid tumor.

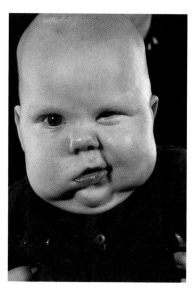

Fig 7-6 Congenital facial paralysis may be due to forceps trauma used at delivery.

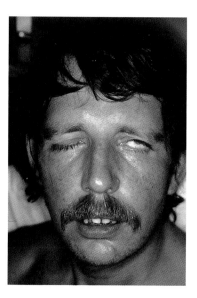

Fig 7-7 Bilateral facial paralysis following head injury. On forced eye closure, the weakness becomes apparent.

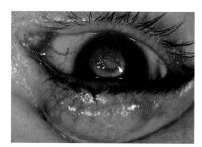

Fig 7-8 Corneal ulceration. This followed exposure keratitis after the onset of facial paralysis. Note the gold weight in the upper lid which is designed to facilitate eye closure.

Care of the eye is the most important consideration in the early management of facial paralysis (Fig 7-8). Without a blink reflex, the cornea is unprotected and may ulcerate. This is particularly so if corneal sensation is impaired (note that the trigeminal and facial nerves are close together at the petrous apex). If in any doubt, early referral to ophthalmology is essential.

It follows that partial paralysis of gradual onset should not be labeled "Bell's palsy." Investigations in such a patient are likely to reveal a specific cause.

Recovery

This depends on the severity of nerve injury. If complete degeneration of the nerve takes place, recovery is likely to be delayed and incomplete. Overall, 90% of patients have satisfactory return

Key Points:

1. All that palsies is not Bell's! The diagnosis of Bell's palsy can only be made by exclusion of other causes of facial paralysis.

2. Protection of the cornea is the most crucial factor in the early management of facial paralysis.

3. Beware of a malignant parotid tumor (remember the deep lobe!) as a cause of facial paralysis.

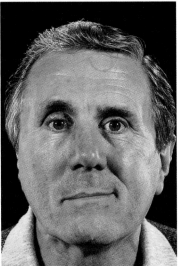

Fig 7-9 Surgical correction of facial paralysis. The patient sustained a fractured temporal bone requiring decompression and repair of the facial nerve. The outcome was an excellent, although imperfect, recovery of facial nerve function.

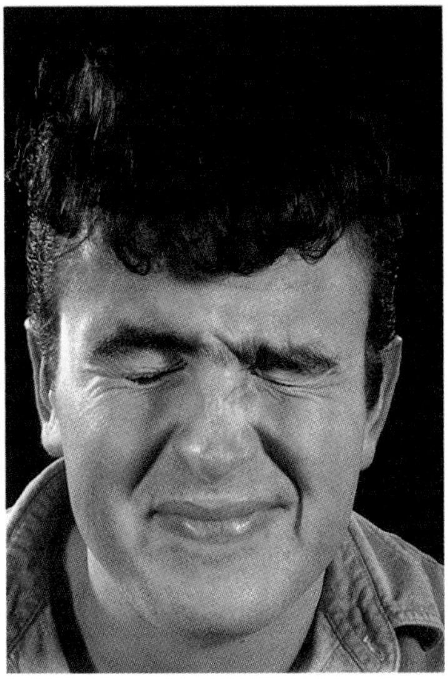

Fig 7-10 Facial nerve surgery. The patient had a dense right facial paralysis following temporal bone fracture. The nerve was explored and a fragment of bone was removed from the nerve. There was almost complete recovery of facial nerve function.

of facial function. Surgery to decompress the nerve is necessary only in exceptional cases.

SURGERY OF THE FACIAL NERVE

The entire facial nerve, from brain stem to the face, is accessible to surgical repair (Figs 7-9 and 7-10). This may involve the combined efforts of an otologist and a neurosurgeon. Microsurgical techniques allow direct end-to-end repair or the interposition of a nerve graft.

Patients whose nerves cannot be repaired in this way can benefit from other techniques that reanimate the paralyzed face. These can improve the patient's appearance, speech, and morale. Patients should be referred to otologists doing such work.

Key Points:

1. The entire facial nerve is amenable to surgical repair.

2. It is possible to reanimate a paralyzed face when the nerve cannot be repaired.

Pediatric Otology

The ear diseases described in previous chapters can all affect children. However, certain conditions occur rather more frequently in children. Hearing impairment also has a different, and possibly greater, impact on children than it does on adults. Speech and language are dependent on good hearing during the critical period of their acquisition, usually the first few years of life. Hearing impairment can also cause developmental delay of motor and social skills and may have profound effects on educational achievement. Hearing is also fundamental to the normal rapport a child has with parents, siblings, and other children. There is thus a sense of urgency about identifying and treating hearing loss in infants and children.

EXAMINATION OF THE EAR IN CHILDREN

Ear examination has been described in Chapter 2. It is essential for the conduct of the examination to have control over both the otoscope and the child. If the child is fractious, as may happen in otitis media, ask the mother or a nurse to hold the child as shown (Fig 8-1). It often helps to let the child see the otoscope and to shine the light on his hand or face before introducing it to the ear. The otoscope should be held like a pen with the examiner's finger on the child's cheek acting as an "early warning system" lest the child should jolt. The pinna should be gently retracted backward to straighten the "S"-shaped canal. If wax obscures the view, it can be syringed or removed with a probe. An instrument must never be introduced into a child's ear canal until the situation is entirely under control. It is better to defer examination rather than risk injuring a child's ear or shattering its confidence.

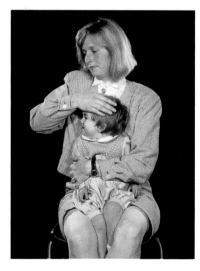

Fig 8-1 Examination of the ear in children. The parent (or nurse) should restrain the child's upper limbs. The lower limbs can be controlled by locking them between the thighs (failure to do so can result in an embarassing injury to the examiner!).

AUDIOLOGICAL ASSESSMENT IN CHILDREN

The most important rule to remember is this: If parents suspect their child has hearing impairment—*believe them!* The younger the child, the more important it is to take stock. Always arrange a formal assessment and, if need be, repeat assessments if doubt continues.

SCREENING AT BIRTH

All children at risk for hearing loss should be screened shortly after birth. The main risk determinants are as shown in Table 8-1.

However, about half the children born with permanent hearing impairments have no known risk factors. To identify these children early in life, universal screening of all children is needed. Until the advent of otoacoustic emissions, this ideal was not achievable because of the practical difficulties involved in testing large numbers of babies (the incidence of permanent hearing impairment is between 1 and 2 per 1000 babies). Otoacoustic emissions are highly sensitive indicators of hearing loss, are noninvasive, and can be used efficiently as a screening tool. Children who fail the screening can either be retested or referred for more definitive testing (behavioral or electrophysiological testing). The importance of early diagnosis lies in the fact that it allows early rehabilitation of these children with hearing aids, and appropriate advice and support can be given to the child's family. Early identification and rehabilitation has been shown to achieve a better long-term outcome when compared to children in whom diagnosis was delayed. Molecular markers of genetic deafness (eg, connexin) may also aid in the early diagnosis of sensorineural deafness.

Parental Suspicion

The importance of heeding parental suspicion cannot be overemphasized. In this context, the myth of the "fussy mother" can safely be buried. In some centers, guidelines are given to every parent of a newborn child. These indicate how babies and infants with normal hearing react to sound. This heightens parental awareness and facilitates early diagnosis, especially in children with no risk factors.

Health Visitor

For most children in the United Kingdom, the first hearing check is performed by the health visitor at between 6 to 8 months of age. The technique used is called *distraction testing*. This requires a cooperative child and considerable skill on the part of the tester. The child usually sits at a table on his parent's lap and his attention is obtained by an observer. The tester introduces a sound surreptitiously from behind the child. The child's reaction is noted by the observer. The results of this type of screening depend on the skill of the health visitor. Alas, many parents of high-risk children (ethnic minorities, low socioeconomic groups) do not attend these clinics or will not bring their children along for definitive testing.

Conditioning Audiometry

From age 18 months to 3½ years a variety of techniques exploit the ability of children of different mental ages to undertake specific

Table 8-1. Causes of Sensorineural Hearing Loss in Childhood

Family history of deafness
Maternal infections: rubella, toxoplasmosis, syphilis, viral infection (cytomegalovirus)
Prematurity
Other congenital abnormalities
Anoxia
Jaundice
Meningitis
Ototoxics (eg, gentamicin)

Key Point:

Otoacoustic emissions are sensitive indicators of hearing loss. They have made universal hearing screening a reality.

Key Point:

Parental suspicion of hearing loss or speech delay should be taken seriously. The myth of the "fussy mom" is obsolete.

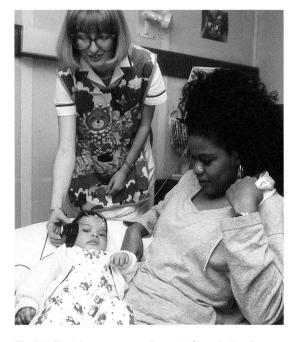

Fig 8-2 Electric response audiometry. Sound stimuli are delivered through a headphone as the child sits on the mother's lap. Recording electrodes are placed on the scalp. The test can be done while the child is asleep on the mother's lap.

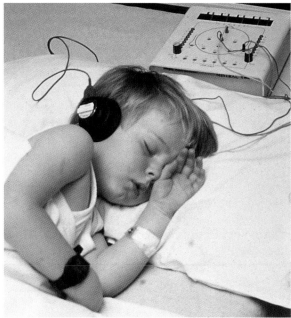

Fig 8-3 Electric response audiometry can also be done on a ward, usually with help of sedation.

tasks. The intensity and frequency of the stimulus can be altered. Given a cooperative child and a skilled tester, a reliable assessment of hearing acuity and discrimination can be obtained.

From about the age of 4 years a pure tone audiogram can be obtained.

Electric Response Audiometry (ERA)

Children with intellectual impairment or behavioral problems may not allow testing by conventional methods. In these children electric response audiometry (see p22) may be necessary to determine hearing levels (Figs 8-2 and 8-3). Occasionally it may be necessary in otherwise normal children where doubt persists after conventional testing. ERA usually requires the child to be either asleep or sedated.

ACUTE SUPPURATIVE OTITIS MEDIA

This is an acute inflammatory process characterized by purulent fluid in the middle ear. It is one of the most common childhood infections. The reasons are poorly understood but are due, at least in part, to the relative immaturity of the eustachian tube and the immune defense mechanisms.

Symptoms

Irritability, progressive throbbing pain, fever, and hearing impairment are the usual symptoms. Untreated, copious purulent discharge from the ear will follow when the eardrum perforates and at this point the pain subsides.

Examination

Be careful–a child with otitis media is usually fractious and will allow only a fleeting glimpse down its ear canal. Sometimes the diagnosis will have to be presumptive. Position the child securely and ensure full control of the otoscope. Inspect behind the pinna for swelling over the mastoid bone (occurs in mastoiditis). The drum will be seen to be hyperemic (Fig 8-4) and often bulging due to pressure from accumulated fluid in the middle ear.

Treatment

Amoxicillin or ampicillin are the preferred initial drugs (the most frequent infecting organisms are *Streptococcus pneumonia* and *Hemophilus influenza*) and should be given for 10 days. If the child is allergic to penicillin, a trimethoprim-sulphamethoxazole combination can be used. Paracetamol is often indicated for pain relief and to lower body temperature. Myringotomy to drain the fluid is rarely done in the UK but is widely practiced in the US. Its advocates find it useful to obtain samples for culture, especially in patients failing to respond to standard antibiotics.

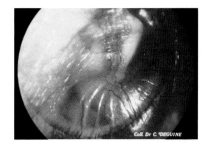

Fig 8-4 Acute otitis media. The tympanic membrane is red and injected with many tiny blood vessels.

> **Key Points:**
> 1. Pain in the ear does not equate with infection. Simple analgesics may be sufficient, especially soon after the onset.
> 2. Antibiotics should only be given when there is evidence of suppuration.
> 3. Ear drops do not have analgesic properties. Oral analgesics are more likely to give pain relief.

RECURRENT OTITIS MEDIA

This can be a most frustrating condition for parents and clinician alike. Parental fatigue from many nights of disturbed sleep is coupled with their anxiety about repeated courses of antibiotics to which they say their child has become "immune."

A search for a nidus of infection elsewhere, eg, sinusitis, is mandatory. An underlying allergy or immune deficiency may need exclusion. Not uncommonly these children have a persistent middle ear effusion which acts as a broth to culture further organisms.

Treatment

It is worth reminding parents of the normal frequency of upper respiratory infection in early childhood to put their child's problem in

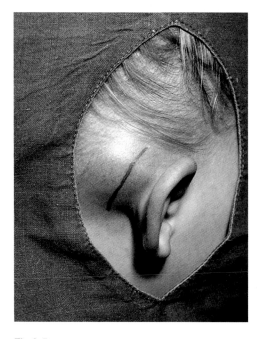

Fig 8-5

Fig 8-6

Fig 8-6 Drainage of the mastoiditis resulted in a free flow of pus (same child as in Fig 8-5).

Fig 8-5 Acute mastoiditis (child aged 3 years). Note the swelling behind the ear pushing the pinna forward. The child is about to have the abscess drained in the operating room.

context. *Prophylactic antibiotics* may be indicated in this situation. This can be continuous low-dose (ie, half the normal therapeutic dose) for a period of 3 to 6 months. Surgery is of limited value in the treatment of recurrent upper respiratory infection. Grommet insertion may be indicated to treat an underlying persistent effusion, especially if hearing impairment compounds the problem.

ACUTE MASTOIDITIS AND MASKED MASTOIDITIS

The incidence of this condition has greatly diminished with the widespread use of antibiotics for otitis media. Antibiotics have made the manner of presentation much more insidious and the danger now is that the diagnosis may go unrecognized. The term "masked" mastoiditis has thus been coined.

Pain and swelling behind the ear are the typical findings. Commonly, the pinna may be pushed forward. The angle the pinna makes with the side of the head may be widened (Figs 8-5 and 8-6). The ear canal is swollen and it is often not possible to see the eardrum. A past history of ear discharge is a helpful pointer.

Untreated, there is a significant risk of intracranial complication (see p40).

Treatment

Requires hospitalization and involves intensive parenteral antibiotics while carefully monitoring the patient's progress. Mastoid exploration may be needed if the situation fails to resolve in 12-24 hours.

OTITIS MEDIA WITH EFFUSION (OME) (CHRONIC SEROUS OTITIS MEDIA, GLUE EAR)

OME has reached epidemic proportions in children in Western countries. It describes a condition characterized by the presence of fluid in the middle ear. As the fluid may be thick and tenacious, the term "glue" ear is often used

Key Points:

1. The possibility of mastoiditis should always be considered if a painful ear fails to respond to therapy.

2. In mastoiditis, examine the patient from behind to assess the forward displacement of the pinna by comparing the protrusion of the right and left ears.

Etiology

Many factors have been implicated: genetic factors, social class, environment, immunity, allergy, eustachian tube insufficiency, sinus infection, and antibiotic treatment of suppurative otitis media. Oxygen is continually being absorbed by the respiratory epithelium resulting in negative pressure in the middle ear. This encourages transudation of fluid from the mucosa.

Symptoms

The highest incidence is in the age group 2 to 5 years. The various modes of presentation may be summarized as follows:

1. *Hearing impairment.* This may fluctuate depending on the volume and consistency of fluid in the middle ear.

2. *Language delay.* The peak incidence of this condition is during the "critical period" for speech and language development.

3. *Behavioral problems.* Because a child cannot hear, he or she is likely to be labeled "disobedient" or "inattentive" both at home and at school. Such children may be described as being detached from their peers and "being in a world of their own."

4. *Recurrent ear infections.* The "glue" is an ideal culture medium for microorganisms.

5. *Reading/learning difficulties at school.*

6. *The "silent syndrome."* A child may be detected with florid serous otitis media purely on screening.

It is important to note that the condition produces hearing impairment at an important period in a child's development, ie, when speech is developing and the child is about to begin school.

Examination

The otoscopic findings are of a dull, featureless, immobile tympanic membrane (Figs 8-7 and 8-8). Sometimes fluid levels can be

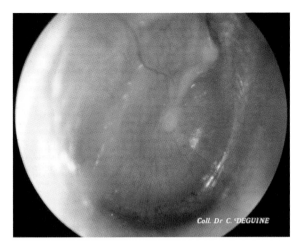

Fig 8-7 Otitis media with effusion (glue ear). This dull, featureless tympanic membrane is very typical of glue ear. Compare with Fig 8-8.

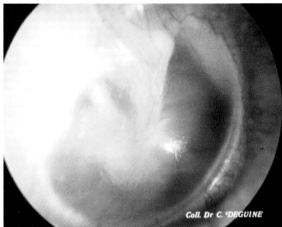

Fig 8-8 A normal tympanic membrane.

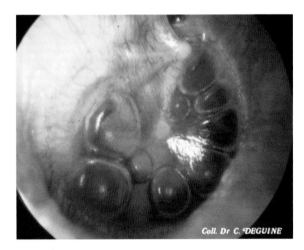

Fig 8-9 Otitis media with effusion (glue ear). Air-fluid levels can be seen behind the tympanic membrane.

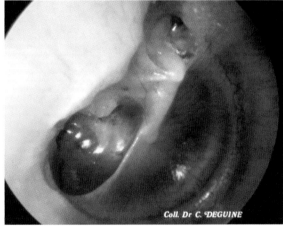

Fig 8-10 Otitis media with effusion (glue ear). Often the tympanic membrane becomes retracted (indrawn) making the lateral process of the malleus more prominent. Note the dull appearance of the drum.

seen (Fig 8-9). Often, the tympanic membrane is indrawn towards the middle ear (retracted) (Fig 8-10).

Treatment

An attempt is made in Table 8-2 to summarize the rationale and shortcomings of some common approaches to the problem.

It is important to bear in mind that about 50% of effusions resolve spontaneously within six weeks of onset. In many instances, a "wait and see" policy is appropriate.

Table 8-2. Treatment Options for OME (Otitis Media With Effusion—"Glue" Ear)

Treatment	Advantage	Disadvantage
No treatment	No risk. Natural history favors spontaneous resolution.	May involve prolonged periods of hearing loss.
Decongestants	Avoids hospitalization.	No proven value. Can cause behavioral disorders. Expensive in long term.
Long-term antibiotics	Avoids hospitalization.	Not a long-term cure. Not all children benefit.
Myringotomy alone	Low risk. Immediate hearing gain. Can be done as day case.	Relief short-lived. Requires anesthesia and hospitalization.
Grommet insertion	As for myringotomy.	Requires anesthesia and hospitalization.
	Relief from hearing loss 6-9 months.	Ear may discharge. Swimming forbidden by some surgeons. May scar eardrum (tympanosclerosis) or cause a perforation.
Adenoidectomy	Improves eustachian tube function. Relieves catarrhal symptoms.	Needs anesthesia and hospitalization. Not usually done as a day case. May bleed post-operatively. Benefit disputed.
Hearing aid	Assures hearing restoration. Avoids surgery.	Parental dislike. Does not prevent the harmful effects of middle ear effusion on the tympanic membrane (atelect)

Ventilating Tubes (Grommets)

Ventilating tubes (grommets) are tiny tubes inserted in the tympanic membrane (Fig 8-11). Their purpose is to promote the ventilation of the middle ear rather than drainage of fluid. Insertion usually results in a dramatic gain in hearing and relief from earache. They remain in position for about 6 to 18 months and are extruded spontaneously by the tympanic membrane.

Ear discharge may follow grommet insertion. This is best treated by dry mopping the ear canal and inserting ear drops. Occasionally systemic antibiotics are necessary. If discharge persists, refer to the ENT department.

Whether or not a child can go swimming is very much dependent on the individual surgeon. Some prohibit swimming

Fig 8-11 Ventilating tubes (grommets). Note that the middle ear is well ventilated.

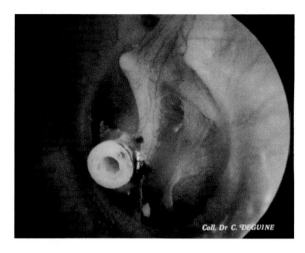

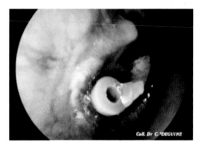

Fig 8-12 Ventilating tubes (grommets) and tympanosclerosis. Following grommet insertion a small horseshoe-shaped ring of tympanosclerosis (white "chalk patches") can form in the tympanic membrane.

completely. A number of studies, however, show that grommets do not increase the likelihood of infection after swimming. Thus, after a period of 2 weeks, some surgeons are happy for their patients to swim, even without earplugs.

Some children require repeated grommet insertion (about 1 in 5 of children requiring surgical treatment) and parents tend to become disillusioned. In such patients, it is imperative that an underlying aggravating cause (eg, allergy, sinus disease, adenoid hypertrophy) is sought and treated. Recurrent or persistent glue ear that defies the usual remedies can be extremely difficult to manage.

Grommets may cause tympanosclerosis (Fig 8-12) of the tympanic membrane but this is generally considered not to affect hearing. Rarely, a tiny perforation (Fig 8-13) may persist after grommet extrusion.

Possible effects of otitis media with effusion on the middle ear are outlined in Table 8-3.

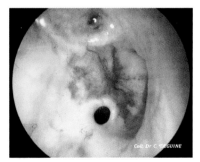

Fig 8-13 Perforation following grommet extrusion. Occasionally a pinhole perforation may persist after extrusion of the tube. This may need surgical repair.

Table 8-3. Possible Otological Sequelae of Otitis Media With Effusion ("Glue Ear").

Atelectasis	A weak, floppy tympanic membrane which tends to be sucked into the middle ear. The drum may get stuck to the ossicles or to the promontory (adhesive otitis). Such thin drums readily perforate.
Retraction pockets	With advancing atelectasis, the eardrum may form pockets, which tend to collect epithelial debris.
Erosion of ossicles	The long process of the incus tends to get eroded in this condition.
Tympanosclerosis	Results from the drum developing calcific changes from repeated infection. It may sometimes follow ventilating tube insertion.
Cholesteatoma	An uncertain association exists between chronic glue ear and cholesteatoma. This may be the result of retraction pocket formation or of metaplastic changes in the middle ear mucosa.

SENSOINEURAL HEARING LOSS

There are two main causes: *Genetic* and *acquired* (prenatal or postnatal).

Genetic

This is overwhelmingly the most important single cause of sensorineural hearing impairment in childhood and may account for more than 50% of permanent cases. The mode of transmission is autosomal recessive in 80% of cases, autosomal dominant in 15%, and x-linked in 2-3%. Most hearing losses are not associated with specific syndromes. The syndromes most often associated with hearing loss are shown in Table 8-4. These syndromes typically have instantly recognizable features, such as the white forelock in Waardenburg's syndrome (Fig 8-14). Markers of genetic deafness (eg, connexin) offer the possibility of early recognition and the hope of therapeutic intervention in the future.

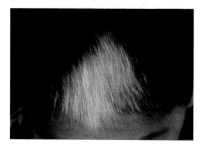

Fig 8-14 Waardenburg's syndrome is characterized by a white forelock and sensorineural hearing loss.

Table 8-4. Some Common Syndromes Associated With Deafness Along With Their Typical Mode of Inheritance

Syndrome	Disorders	Mode of Inheritance
Waardenburg's syndrome	Pigmentary abnormalities (hair, eyes, etc.)	Autosomal dominant
Usher syndrome	Retinitis pigmentosa	Autosomal recessive
Pendred's syndrome	Thyroid dysfunction	Autosomal recessive
Alport syndrome	Renal insufficiency	Variable inheritance
Neurofibromatosis, type 2	Bilateral acoustic tumors, other intracranial tumors	Autosomal dominant
Treacher Collins syndrome	Mandibulofacial abnormalities	Autosomal dominant

Key Point:
Genetic factors have a major role to play in permanent hearing impairment and should be routinely sought in the assessment of childhood deafness.

Acquired

Prenatal

Certain infections acquired *in utero* can affect the developing auditory system (eg, rubella, cytomegalovirus, syphilis).

Postnatal

Bacterial meningitis, which has a very high incidence in the first 2 years of life, is the most important cause. About 1% of children with meningitis will have profound bilateral sensorineural hearing loss.

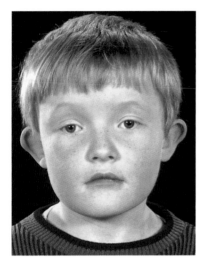

Fig 8-15 Bilateral "bat" ears.

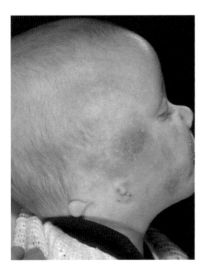

Fig 8-16 Microtia. This child was born with major malformation of the external and middle ears.

Management

Crucially important in management is early and accurate diagnosis. Only then can appropriate rehabilitative measures be instituted. The most important factor in rehabilitation is the early fitting of appropriate hearing aids which can be fitted in the first few months of life. Access to high quality speech and language therapy is particularly important in the early years. Parents and family need counselling to understand the implications of profound deafness and advice on how best to facilitate the development of speech and language. Such counselling is particularly important as over 90% of deaf children are born to normally hearing parents who may have little prior exposure to deafness. Genetic counselling should always be offered to parents.

Special arrangements for the child's education need to be made depending on the severity of the hearing loss. Some will attend mainstream school wearing their hearing aids. Those requiring more help will need the services of a Partial Hearing Unit in the UK or Special Education in the US. Special residential schools may be necessary for those with total or near total deafness. There is no unanimity about which educational environment is optimal for the deaf child and much may depend on educational policy where the child lives.

CONGENITAL DEFORMITIES OF THE EAR

"Bat" Ears

Abnormally protruding ears can make a child the object of derision from his peers and cause emotional problems (Fig 8-15). Therefore, the deformity ought to be corrected before school age, ie, about the age of 5 years. The operation of pinnaplasty permanently "pins back" the offending ears.

Congenital Deformity of the Pinna (Microtia)

The severity of this deformity is variable (Fig 8-16). Sometimes the pinna may be absent or rudimentary. These deformities are often associated with an absent ear canal and middle ear. Fortunately, the inner ear is nearly always normal due to its totally different embryological development. Hence, it is essential that these children have their hearing assessed and hearing aids fitted at the earliest possible opportunity. Treacher Collins syndrome is a combination of multiple facial deformities with abnormalities of the pinna and middle ear.

Treatment

The results of multiple plastic surgical procedures to reconstruct the pinnae on these children have been disappointing. Children

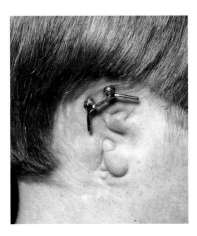

Fig 8-17 Osseointegration. Titanium screws can be fixed in the mastoid bone to provide anchorage for a prosthetic pinna.

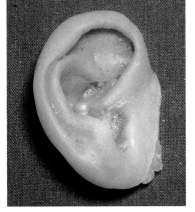

Fig 8-18 The prosthetic pinna.

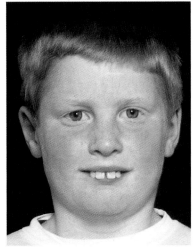

Fig 8-19 Osseointegration. The end result (compare with Fig 8-17). This technology saves the trauma and disappointment of conventional techniques of pinna reconstruction. A hearing aid can also be anchored in bone at the same time (see Figs 9-5 and 9-6).

and their parents can now be spared this trauma thanks to advances in osseointegrated implants (Figs 8-17–8-19). Not only does this result in a superior cosmetic result but a bone-anchored hearing aid can also be implanted in bilateral cases (see Figs 9-2 and 9-3 in the next chapter).

> **Key Point:**
> Bone-anchored technology can be used to fix an artificial pinna or to maintain a bone-conducting hearing aid.

Preauricular Sinuses

These are due to incomplete fusion of the primitive tubercles that form the pinna (Fig 8-20). They can cause troublesome discharge and are often more extensive than they at first appears. Treatment is surgical removal.

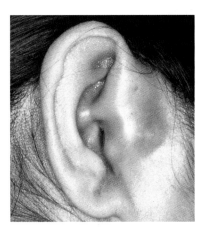

Fig 8-20 Infected preauricular sinus. This is due to incomplete fusion of the hillocks that form the ear. Note the tiny pit, which is always present.

Hearing Aids, Cochlear Implants, and Tinnitus Maskers

HEARING AIDS

In the UK, over 200 000 hearing aids are issued in the UK by the National Health Service (NHS) annually. With an aging population in most Western countries, these figures are likely to rise even higher. Hearing aids function by selectively amplifying sound. They work best for conductive losses because inner ear function is usually normal and the problem is purely one of sound amplification. They are thus ideal in otosclerosis or stable chronic ear disease. In general, the better the inner ear function, the more efficiently the hearing aid will work. Thus, given a choice between two ears with hearing impairment, it is usually best to fit the aid on the "good" ear. This often comes as a surprise to the patient!

Components

Hearing aids have four components: a miniature microphone; an amplifier, a receiver, and a mold.

The *microphone* picks up the incoming sound.

The *amplifier* makes the sound louder.

The *receiver* feeds the sound into the ear.

The *mold* is worn in the external ear.

Limitations

Hearing aids amplify sounds. This means that background noise (usually low frequency) is also amplified, which can interfere significantly with speech intelligibility. Patients with good low-frequency but poor high-frequency hearing are most troubled by this. Some patients with impaired cochlear function are exquis-

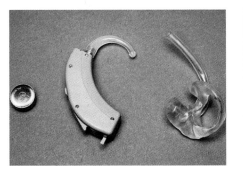

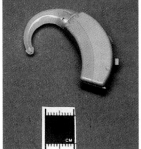

Fig 9-1

Fig 9-2

Fig 9-1 Behind-the-ear (BTE) hearing aid assembly. The hearing aid is connected to a mold (on the right), which is inserted in the ear canal. The mold is individually made for each patient so as to obtain a comfortable fit. These aids are powered by small batteries (left).

Fig 9-2 Behind-the-ear aid—"micro." This tiny device can be fitted to babies a few months old.

itely sensitive to noise (a phenomenon called *recruitment*) and getting these patients to benefit from hearing aids may be difficult or impossible.

Some patients find hearing aids either cosmetically or socially unacceptable. They feel it draws attention to their disability, which they wish to hide, but modern miniaturized aids have done a lot to reduce this. Others feel hearing aids are stigmatizing, associated with old age, and make them less competitive in the workplace.

Hearing aids need an insert (mold) in the ear canal and this can cause otitis externa. The precise fitting of an earmold is of crucial importance and requires considerable care. Hearing aids cannot be worn in discharging ears.

Digitally programmable hearing aids have been a major advance and offer greater flexibility with hearing aid fitting than was previously possible.

Hearing Therapy

It must be emphasized that the provision of a hearing aid marks the beginning of a rehabilitation program. Alas, many patients reject their hearing aids because of inadequate counselling and support. Some deafened patients may be utterly dejected by their disability, especially when their employment is threatened. Enabling patients with multiple handicaps to use hearing aids successfully is a major challenge. Hearing therapists advise on lip reading, environmental aids, hearing aid skills, and undertake auditory training, and their services should be sought in appropriate cases.

Hearing Aid Types

Behind-the-Ear (BTE)

These aids are the most commonly prescribed by the National Health Service in the UK (Figs 9-1 and 9-2). They can be quite powerful and are generally cosmetically acceptable. Adjusting the settings needs a certain amount of manual dexterity and can be a problem in the elderly, especially those with arthritis or neurological disability.

Body Worn (BW)

These aids may be necessary for patients with profound hearing losses or those who do not have the manipulative skills to manage a "behind the ear" aid. The microphone is on the device and the patient's clothing may impair the sound uptake. Friction between the clothes and the microphone can also be annoying.

"In-the-Ear" (ITE) and "In-the-Canal" (ITC) Aids

These aids (Figs 9-3 and 9-4) are accommodated entirely in the external ear. They are suitable for mild to moderate hearing losses. They are cosmetically more acceptable than the behind-the-ear variety but are costly.

Bone-Anchored Aids

These have supplanted the conventional bone conducting aids, which were fixed by means of a headband. The bone anchored aids are fixed by means of a special titanium screw in the mastoid bone and are highly efficient sound conductors (Figs 9-5 and 9-6). They are most useful in congenital ear abnormalities where there may be no pinna on which to hang an ordinary aid. They

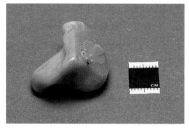

Fig 9-4 In-the-canal (ITE) aid. These sophisticated devices fit in the ear canal and are cosmetically acceptable.

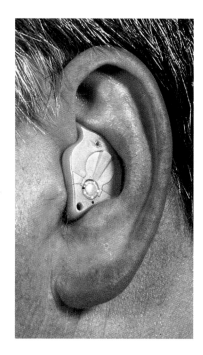

Fig 9-3 In-the-ear (ITC) hearing aid. The attractiveness of these aids is readily apparent. The part that is inserted in the ear canal is shown on the right.

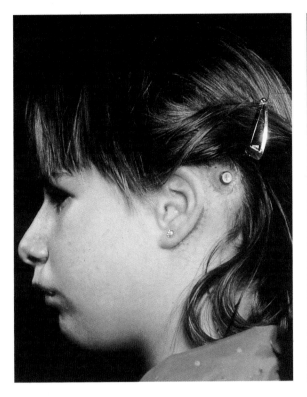

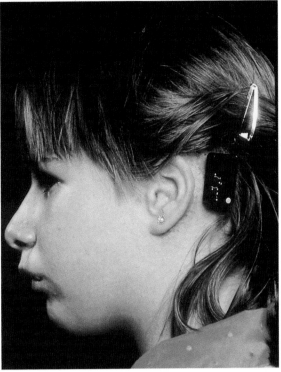

Fig 9-5 Bone-anchored aid. These are necessary when the patient has no pinna or is unable to wear conventional hearing aids (eg, due to atresia of the ear canal). The first stage is the insertion of a titanium screw, which becomes anchored solidly in bone.

Fig 9-6 Bone-anchored aid. The aid is clipped on the screw that transmits the sound vibration through bone to the cochlea.

can also be extremely useful in those patients with intractable discharging ears who are intolerant of earmolds in their ear canals.

Implantable Hearing Aids

The desire to develop hearing aids that are totally implanted stems from the wishes of many patients not to wear any external equipment that draws attention to their disability. The technological challenges posed by such systems are considerable and, as yet, there are no systems in routine clinical use.

Key Points:

1. The provision of a hearing aid marks the beginning of a rehabilitation program to improve communication skills.

2. Always fully examine the ears in a patient with hearing loss. Any suspicion of underlying disease requires referral to ENT (remember acoustic neuroma, etc).

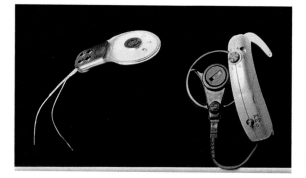

Fig 9-7 a

Fig 9-7 a. Cochlear implant. On the left is the portion that is implanted at surgery; on the right is the ear-level transmitter coil and the speech processor. **b.** The electrodes are inserted into the spiral of the cochlea to stimulate the surviving auditory nerve endings.

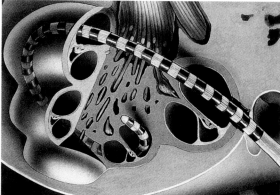

Fig 9-7 b

COMMERCIAL VS. NHS HEARING AIDS

In the UK, hearing aids are available free of charge from the NHS. Commercial aids can be very costly. The maintenance (repairs, batteries, etc) of NHS aids is carried out without charge to the patient. Financial considerations are especially important to the elderly who may no longer be in employment and for whom the cost of a commercial aid may need to be met out of savings. A wider selection of very sophisticated aids is available commercially, especially in-the-ear varieties which are prescribed only for special medical reasons by the NHS.

Patients opting to buy hearing aids should be advised to see a reputable dealer and insist on a free trial of the device in their everyday environment. This may mean trying several aids. The patient should be advised against judging the value of an aid on its performance in the acoustically ideal environment of a sound-treated room.

The greatest criticisms of NHS aids are the time delay between referral for assessment and fitting of the device and the limited choice of instruments.

COCHLEAR IMPLANTS

Cochlear implants ("bionic ears") represent a breakthrough in the management of acquired total deafness. These patients derive little or no benefit from even the most powerful hearing aids. The deafness may have been acquired (eg, due to meningitis, ototoxic medications, or head injury) or may be congenital.

The system consists of an ear level microphone which collects sound. A body-worn or ear level speech processor converts the sound to electrical signals. These signals are then passed to electronic circuitry implanted at the time of surgery. Tiny electrodes convey the signals directly to the auditory nerve (Figs 9-7, a and b), thus bypassing the function of the cochlea.

In congenitally deaf children, cochlear implants provide the best results when implanted early in life, usually before the age of 5 years. There is a trend toward earlier implantation as the auditory system seems most receptive to electrical stimulation early in life. Children who lose their hearing (usually due to meningitis) are best implanted as soon as possible after the onset of deafness (Fig 9-8). There is the additional concern following meningitis that new bone can form in the cochlea thus making implantation more difficult. Adults who are deafened after acquiring spoken language are excellent implant candidates and the earlier the intervention is undertaken the better.

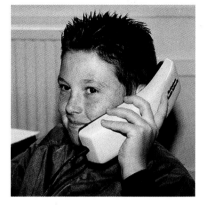

Fig 9-8 Cochlear implant. This child was totally deafened following a head injury. He received a cochlear implant and subsequently developed the ability to communicate over the telephone.

Key Points:

1. Cochlear implants are *indicated* in patients who derive little or no benefit from hearing aids.

2. Congenitally deaf children should be implanted early in life to get the best results.

3. Children who lose their hearing, especially following meningitis, should be referred urgently to an implant center before the cochlea is obliterated by new bone formation.

TINNITUS MASKERS

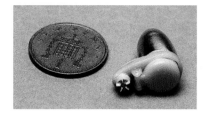

Fig 9-9 Tinnitus masker. This device is worn in the ear canal and can produce a sound similar to the patient's tinnitus. This has the effect of masking or "drowning" the indigenous noise.

The rationale for this approach is to use an extraneous noise which drowns out or "masks" the noise of the tinnitus. This gives the patient a sense of control over the symptom. It follows that the patient's tinnitus must be of such a quality as to allow this matching to take place. Tinnitus that varies in quality or is very bizarre may be impossible to mask. Maskers are worn like hearing aids (Fig 9-9). They are not a "cure" for tinnitus and should only be used as part of a comprehensive rehabilitation program.

PART 2

The Nose and Sinuses

CHAPTER 10

Clinical Anatomy and Physiology

ANATOMY OF THE NOSE

The External Nose

The nasal skeleton consists of the nasal bones, the paired lateral cartilages, and the septal cartilage (Fig 10-1). The proportion of the nose made up by the nasal bones varies between 30% and 70%. Each nasal bone is attached to the frontal bone and the maxilla. Trauma to the nose can fracture the nasal bones which may be deviated or depressed.

There are paired upper and lower lateral (alar) cartilages. Each upper lateral cartilage is attached to the under surface of the nasal bone and to the nasal septum. The septum, therefore, provides support to the dorsum of the nose. The delicate lower lateral cartilages are responsible for the support and appearance of the nasal tip. The shape of the nasal bones and cartilages has a bearing both on the appearance and the function of the nose.

The arterial supply to the external nose comes from branches of the facial and ophthalmic arteries. These vessels may bleed significantly after facial trauma. The angular vein lies at the medial canthus and it is via this vein that infection of the face can spread to the cavernous sinus. The angular vein may be damaged during rhinoplasty and this can result in bruising (black eyes). The lymphatic vessels of the external nose drain to the upper deep cervical chain.

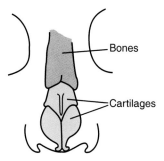

Fig 10-1 The nasal skeleton consists of 2 nasal bones, 2 pairs of lateral cartilages (upper and lower), and the septal cartilage.

The Nasal Cavity

The septum divides the nasal cavity into two halves. The floor of the nasal cavity runs in a horizontal direction, parallel with the hard palate. The vestibule is the skin-covered area at the entrance of each nostril. Hairs cover part of the vestibular skin so that a furuncle may arise in this region. The nasal valve is the narrowest portion of the nostril and demarcates the vestibule from the nasal cavity proper. The columella is the strut at the caudal end of the septum between the two nostrils.

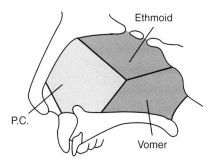

Fig 10-2 The septum consists of the quadrilateral cartilage and the vomer and ethmoid bones.

The Septum

The septum, which supports the dorsum of the nose, consists of the quadrilateral cartilage joined to the vomer and the ethmoid bones (Fig 10-2).

The Lateral Wall of the Nose

The lateral wall of the nose has 3 projecting shelves of bone known as turbinates or conchae (Fig 10-3). These serve to increase the surface area of the nasal cavity. The turbinates are labeled superior, middle, and inferior and the space under each turbinate is called a meatus (Fig 10-4).

The middle meatus lies under the middle turbinate and is the most important functional area. All the sinuses open into this meatus with the exception of the sphenoid and posterior ethmoidal cells. The openings of the sinus ostia into the middle meatus are close together and form the *ostio-meatal complex* (Fig 10-5). This is a key area because pathology in this region can interfere with ventilation and mucociliary clearance of the sinuses.

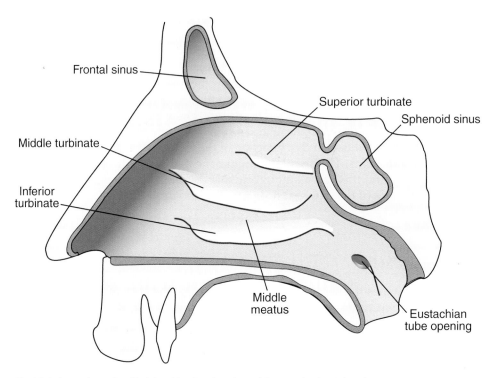

Fig 10-3 Lateral nasal wall, right side showing the turbinates, the frontal and sphenoid sinus. Adapted with permission from *American Family Physician*. 1998;58(3):712. Copyright 1998 by American Family Physician.

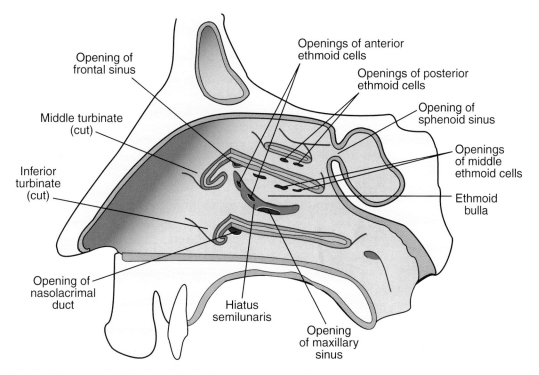

Fig 10-4 Lateral wall right side with turbinates removed shows the openings into the frontal ethmoid and maxillary sinuses. Reprinted with permission from *American Family Physician* 1998;58(3):712. Copyright 1998 by American Family Physician.

Fiberoptic endoscopes allow the surgeon to inspect and operate on the ostio-meatal complex.

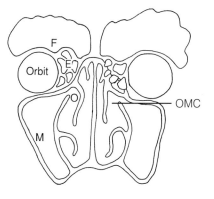

Key Points:

1. All the sinuses with the exception of the posterior ethmoidal cells and the sphenoid sinus open into the middle meatus.

2. The ostiomeatal complex in the middle meatus is the key area for endoscopic sinus surgery.

3. Only one structure, the nasolacrimal duct, opens into the inferior meatus.

Fig 10-5 Coronal section of the sinuses. The cilia direct the mucus out of the sinus ostia. Note the paper-thin bone between the ethmoid sinuses and the orbit know as the lamina papyracea. F = frontal sinus, E = Ethmoids, O = sinus ostia, M = maxillary, OMC = Ostio-meatal complex.

Epithelial Lining of the Nasal Cavity

There are 2 types of epithelium within the nose: olfactory and respiratory.

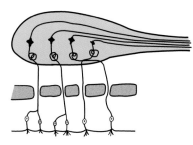

Fig 10-6 The olfactory epithelium lines the superior part of the nose. The filaments of the olfactory nerve are vulnerable to injury as they pass through the cribriform plate.

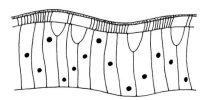

Fig 10-7 The pseudostratified ciliated columnar epithelium, know as respiratory epithelium, lines the nose, sinuses, trachea, and bronchi. Mucociliary action keeps the respiratory tract moist and clean. Small hooks on the end of the cilia pull the viscous gel layer forward during the effective stroke. The recovery stroke occurs mainly in the thin sol layer.

Key Points:

1. Because of their relatively large size, the ethmoid sinuses are particularly important in children.

2. The ethmoid sinuses are intimately related with the orbit, the cribriform plate and the optic nerve.

3. Nasal polyps originate from the ethmoid air cells.

Olfactory Epithelium

This is confined to the superior part of the nasal cavity (Fig 10-6). It extends medially to the septum and laterally onto the superior turbinate. Olfactory epithelium is nonciliated and contains the bipolar olfactory cells. The axons of these neurons combine into about 20 olfactory nerves, which pass through the cribriform plate to relay in the olfactory bulb. Trauma to the cribriform plate may shear the olfactory neurons resulting in loss of smell.

Respiratory Epithelium

This epithelium lines the rest of the nasal cavity (Fig 10-7). It is a pseudostratified, ciliated columnar epithelium. The respiratory epithelium which lines the nose and sinuses is the same as that lining the trachea, bronchi, and eustachian tube. Goblet cells and mucous glands are distributed throughout the submucosa.

ANATOMY OF THE SINUSES

The sinuses are bony cavities within the skull. They are all formed as diverticula from the nasal cavity and are, therefore, lined with respiratory epithelium. The sinuses consist of the paired frontal sinuses and maxillary sinuses (antra), and finally the spenoid sinuses.

The Ethmoid Sinuses

The ethmoid sinuses (see Fig 10-5) lie between the orbits and comprise a labyrinth of about 20 intercommunicating air cells. Nasal polyps arise from the ethmoid sinuses. A polyp may originate from each ethmoid cell which explains why they are often multiple. The ethmoid sinuses are particularly important in childhood where they account for a large proportion of the facial skeleton.

Relations. The lateral wall of the ethmoid sinus is paper thin and is consequently known as the lamina papyracea. Infection in the ethmoid sinus may spread through the lamina papyracea into the orbit. The roof of the ethmoid sinus is called the cribriform plate and it forms part of the floor of the anterior cranial fossa. Trauma to the cribriform plate often results in a cerebrospinal fluid (CSF) leak. Spread of infection or tumor to the anterior cranial fossa can occur through the ethmoid roof or via the ethmoidal vessels. Posteriorly the ethmoid cells lie close to the apex of the orbit and the optic nerve.

The Maxillary Sinus (Antrum)

This is the largest sinus, with a volume of 15–30 ml (see Fig 10-5). Rudimentary at birth, the sinus grows quickly with the secondary dentition and eventually the floor of the sinus lies below the floor of the nose. Mucus and debris cannot be cleared from the sinus by gravity but rely on the action of the cilia. These cilia direct the mucus through the sinus ostia, which is high up on the medial wall and opens into the middle meatus.

The roots of the premolar and first molar teeth may project into the antrum and consequently dental infection may lead to secondary sinus infection. Following dental extraction, an oro-antral fistula may arise.

Relations. The roof of the sinus forms the floor of the orbit. The infraorbital nerve runs across the roof and the bone covering it may be dehiscent. Fractures that involve the sinus roof may, therefore, lead to trapping of orbital contents or damage to the infraorbital nerve. The posterior wall of the sinus separates the antrum from the pterygopalatine fossa. The maxillary artery lies in the pterygopalatine fossa and access to this artery can be gained through the maxillary sinus.

Frontal Sinuses

The frontal sinuses (see Fig 10-5) develop from the recess in the anterior part of the nose. They are rudimentary before the age of 7 years. Pneumatization into the frontal bone then occurs and its extent is extremely variable. The frontal sinuses are extensions of the ethmoid air cells.

The frontoethmoidal recess is an "hourglass"-shaped narrowing between the anterior ethmoid cells and the frontal sinus. Trauma, inflammation, mucoceles, and osteomata may obstruct the frontoethmoidal recess and cause frontal sinusitis.

The front wall of the sinus is diploeic bone, which allows infection to track within the 2 layers. Osteomyelitis may follow frontal sinusitis and produce the Pott's puffy tumor (see Fig 15-5).

Relations. Only a thin posterior wall separates the sinus from the frontal lobe and this may provide a route for the intracranial spread of infection. Fractures can also breach this posterior wall. The floor of the sinus is the roof of the orbit.

The Sphenoid Sinuses

The sphenoid sinuses lie in the body of the sphenoid bone, which is quite literally in the center of the head. The sinus is present at birth but is rudimentary. Pneumatization occurs from 10 years onward and is extremely variable. The trans-sphenoidal route is a common approach for pituitary surgery and limited pneumatization makes this surgical approach more difficult. The ostia of the sphenoid sinus is on the anterior wall and it opens directly into the posterior nose.

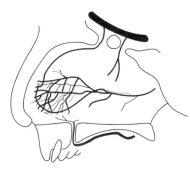

Fig 10-8 Arterial blood supply of the nose. The superior part of the nose is supplied by the internal carotid and the inferior part of the nose by the external carotid.

Key Points:

1. The blood supply of the nose comes from both internal and external carotid systems.

2. The sphenopalatine artery is the most important artery and can be ligated in patients with severe epistaxis.

3. The veins of the nose, face, and sinuses have intracranial communications, which may act as routes for the spread of infection (eg, cavernous sinus thrombosis, meningitis, frontal lobe abscess).

Relations. The lateral wall of the sinus separates it from the cavernous venous sinus whose contents include cranial nerves III-VI. The internal carotid artery also lies in the lateral wall of the cavernous sinus. During pituitary surgery, this fact is important because it is essential to stay in the midline when penetrating the anterior wall of the pituitary fossa as there is only 4 to 8 mm between the two internal carotid arteries at this point.

Blood Supply to the Nose and Sinuses

The nose and sinuses are supplied by both the *external and internal carotid arteries* (Fig 10-8).

The Sphenopalatine Artery (supplies 90%)

The sphenopalatine artery enters the lateral wall of the nose through the sphenopalatine foramen. This lies behind the ostium of the maxillary sinus. The sphenopalatine artery is the most important artery supplying the nose. It is a branch of the maxillary artery, which in turn comes off the external carotid. In patients with persistent epistaxis, the sphenopalatine artery can be ligated.

The Anterior and Posterior Ethmoid Arteries (supplies 10%)

These are branches of the ophthalmic artery, which in turn is a branch of the internal carotid artery, and supply the superior part of the nose. The anterior ethmoid artery passes across the roof of the nose immediately behind the frontoethmoidal recess. It can occasionally cause troublesome bleeding during endoscopic surgery.

Venous Drainage

The venous drainage of the nose and sinuses is provided by the ophthalmic and facial veins and the pterygoid and pharyngeal plexuses. The venous drainage is, therefore, both intracranial and extracranial. The intracranial connection is important because infections of the face can drain via these drains to the cavernous sinus.

Littles' Area (Kiesselbach's Plexus) (see Fig 18-1)

This is an area where several vessels anastomose on the anterior septum. It is a frequent site of epistaxis.

Nerve Supply to the Nose and Sinuses

The nose and sinuses receive sensory, special sensory (smell) and autonomic nerve supplies.

Sensory

The sensory nerve supply is provided by the first and second branches of the trigeminal nerve.

Special Sensory (Olfactory)

The first order neurons are bipolar cells, the axons of which pass through the cribriform plate and relay at the olfactory bulb (see Fig 10-6). The neurons from the bulb run in the olfactory tract to the secondary olfactory center in the frontal lobe. The cortical olfactory center is in the dentate and semilunate gyri.

Autonomic

The autonomic nerve supply provides secretomotor and vasomotor control. Sympathetic fibers arise from the first 5 thoracic segments of the spinal cord. The fibers synapse in the superior cervical ganglion and the post ganglionic fibers run with the blood vessels to the nose and sinuses. An increase in sympathetic tone causes vasoconstriction and decreased secretion.

The parasympathetic supply to the nose is from the lacrimal nucleus with the fibers leaving the brain stem in the nervus intermedius. They relay in the pterygopalatine ganglion before entering the nasal cavity. An increase in parasympathetic tone causes swelling and increased secretion from the nasal mucosa. The pterygopalatine ganglion is sometimes called the "hay fever ganglion."

The Lymphatic Drainage of Nose and Sinuses

The front of the nose and the anterior sinuses drain to the submandibular lymph nodes and then to the deep cervical chain. The back of the nose and the posterior sinuses drain to the retropharyngeal lymph nodes and then to the jugular nodes.

PHYSIOLOGY OF THE NOSE AND SINUSES

The nose is an organ of special sense and respiration. It is an air conditioner so that clean, warm, moist air is provided to the lungs. The nose, sinuses, and lungs should be thought of as one physiological unit. The nose is also important in the production of sound.

Respiration

A newborn baby can only breathe nasally. If both nostrils are blocked (choanal atresia), an oral airway is required if the child is to survive. A relative dependence on nasal respiration continues into adult life, so that mouth breathing should only occur with exertion.

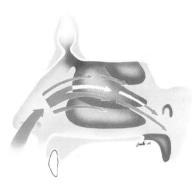

Fig 10-9 Inspiratory airflow. The flow is laminar and occurs primarily over the middle turbinate.

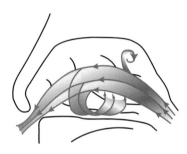

Fig 10-10 Expiratory airflow. Note the turbulence.

The nasal valve is the narrowest part of the nose. The nasal valve lies at the junction of the upper and lower lateral cartilages. The speed of the airstream at the valve is fast and the resistance to flow is high. On inspiration, most of the air passes through the central part of the nasal cavity, up alongside the middle turbinates (Fig 10-9). On expiration the airstream demonstrates turbulence (Fig 10-10).

The Nose as an Air Conditioner

The nose warms, humidifies, and cleans the inspired air.

Heat Exchange

As the air passes over the warm nasal mucosa, it extracts heat. By the time it reaches the nasopharynx, the temperature of the inspired air ranges between 30° and 34°C and is independent of the external temperature. If the external temperature falls, more blood is diverted to the nose so that the cavernous spaces within the mucosa and nasal turbinates swell. The heat output from the nose therefore increases. The reverse situation occurs when the ambient temperature rises. There is a standing temperature gradient from the front of the nose to the back, so that on expiration heat is returned to the nose.

Humidification

Even if an individual is breathing dry desert air, the nose is able to humidify the air so that when it reaches the nasopharynx it is 85% saturated. By the time the inspired air reaches the alveoli it is between 95% and 100% saturated.

Cleaning

The nose also cleans the inspired air. Particles over 4 micromillimeters are filtered by the nose and removed in the mucus. Smaller particles pass on to the lung and are then removed by macrophages.

The Protective Function of the Nose

The protective function of the nose is intimately related to its air-conditioning function. By cleaning and humidifying the air, the respiratory tract is protected. In addition, defense is provided by the mucus blanket, immunoglobulins, and the full range of immune cells.

The Mucous Blanket

This has 2 layers: a gel and sol phase. The top gel layer has a high viscosity and it is this layer that is moved by the ciliary beat. Each cilium is approximately 5 μm long and 0.3 μm thick and consists of microtubules arranged in a 9 × 2 pattern (Fig 10-11). The recovery stroke of the cilia occur mainly in the low viscosity sol layer. Movement of the cilia is like a wheat field swaying on a windy day so that all the cilia do not move at once.

The mucous blanket moves backwards from the front of the nose to the postnasal space in about 20 minutes. In patients with Kartagener's syndrome, no mucociliary transport occurs because the cilia lack dynein arms. These arms contain the adenosine triphosphate that powers the cilia.

Mucociliary transport also occurs throughout the sinuses.

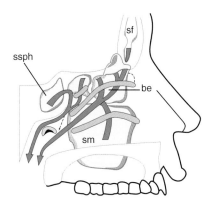

Fig 10-11 Mucociliary pathways. sf = frontal sinus; sm = maxililary sinus; be = ethmoidal bulla; ssph = sphenoid sinus.

Immunological Factors

The submucosa contains lymphocytes, eosinophils, mast cells, and macrophages. IgA, IgM, and IgG are also present in the nasal mucosa. In addition, cells that secrete lysozymes, interferon, and complement factors are present.

Special Sense: Olfaction

Although poorly developed in human beings, a sense of smell adds enormously to the quality of life. The tongue taste buds allow an individual to distinguish between sweet, sour, bitter, and salt. The nuances of taste are provided by the sense of smell. A loss of the sense of smell makes eating and drinking a boring experience! As well as providing pleasurable sensations, the olfactory neurons can also detect unpleasant smells and therefore noxious substances (eg, smoke fumes, gas, etc). Anosmics should be advised to fit smoke detectors.

Only volatile substances can be detected by the olfactory neurons. The molecules of these substances must be soluble in water and lipids, and about 10 to 15 molecules per mm^3 are sufficient to stimulate the olfactory neurons. The sense of smell becomes fatigued so that after a short exposure the subject may be no longer aware of the aroma.

Speech

In speech the nose acts as a variable resonance chamber. The palate shuts the nasopharynx when vowels are formed and opens when consonants are formed. These consonants (eg, m, n, and ng) can be used to test the degree of nasal patency. Nasal obstruction produces a hyponasal voice (eg, the adenoidal child or the patient with nasal polyps).

Nasal Reflexes

In addition to the changes in response to climatic variation, the resistance to breathing in each nostril is continually changing. At any one time one nostril tends to be blocked and the other clear. This alternating pattern is known as the *nasal cycle* and occurs over a 2- to 4-hour period. Other reflexes exist so that if a person sleeps on the right side, the right nostril tends to block and vice versa. Trigeminal nerve endings are present in the nose and are responsible for a diving reflex whereby the heart rate is slowed when the nose contacts cold water (try it!).

Key Points:

1. Mucociliary transport is crucial for nasal function and occurs throughout the nose and sinuses.

2. The nose warms, humidifies and cleanses the inspired air. It is an organ of special sense (smell) and is important in speech production.

3. The nose and lungs should be considered as one functional unit.

4. Anosmics should be advised to fit smoke detectors.

CHAPTER 11

History and Examination

....

HISTORY

There are 6 main symptoms of nasal disease: (1) obstruction, (2) a runny nose and postnasal drip, (3) loss of smell, (4) sneezing, (5) facial pain, and (6) cosmetic deformities.

Obstruction

It is often necessary to ask directly if the patient has difficulty breathing through the nose. The obstruction may be caused by rhinitis; in which case it may be intermittent (seasonal, eg, hay fever) or permanent (perennial rhinitis, eg, house dust mite allergy). Nasal obstruction may be provoked by contact with pollens, molds, pets, dust mites, or other antigens. Alcohol or cigarette smoke may interfere with vasomotor control and lead to obstruction. There may be a coexisting infective element as the hypertrophied allergic mucosa can obstruct the sinus ostia.

Mechanical factors (eg, septal deviations, pneumatized turbinates) are a common cause of nasal obstruction. Nasal obstruction that alternates from one side to the other occurs when the normal *nasal cycle* becomes apparent. A blocked nose leads to mouth breathing and a dry throat. The patient often complains of a sore throat in the morning.

The subjective awareness of nasal blockage varies considerably between individuals and does not always correlate with the assessement made on examination or with special tests.

Runny Nose

A discharge may be clear, yellow, green, or bloodstained.

Green mucopus implies infection but yellow discoloration may be due to eosinophils and allergy.

A unilateral discharge in a child is usually due to a foreign body.

A unilateral discharge in an adult may herald a malignancy, especially if it is bloodstained.

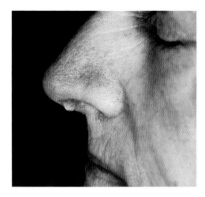

Fig 11-1 Cerebrospinal fluid rhinorrhea. Note its position just under the tip of the nose—not on the nasal floor.

The patient may describe a clear discharge with the nose "running like a tap," which is typical of allergic rhinitis. Rarely, a clear discharge may be due to a leakage of CSF (Fig 11-1).

Most types of rhinosinusitis are accompanied by a nasal discharge. This is usually bilateral and varies from clear to purulent, depending on the extent of infection. Chronic sinus infections are often caused by anaerobic bacteria and the patient may complain of a foul taste or "drainlike" smell.

Crusting within the nose is an unusual symptom and may be associated with granulomatous disease within the nose (eg, Wegener's, sarcoidosis (p163).

In addition to discharge from the front of the nose, patients may complain of a "postnasal drip" or catarrh. It is normal for mucus to be moved backward into the postnasal space where it is swallowed. However, when there is an increased quantity of nasal secretions resulting from infection a foul-tasting drip at the back of the nose develops.

Beware of the persistent unilateral nasal discharge.

Smell

Ask if the loss of smell is total or not.

Frequently a patient may complain of "a complete loss of smell" when there is merely a reduction in smell (hyposmia). Partial loss of smell makes it likely that there is no significant damage to the olfactory nerve and that the primary problem is rhinitis or polyps, both of which are treatable. Smell and taste are closely related so that a reduction in the sense of smell may lead the patient to complain of a "loss of taste." Hyposmia may occur with acute rhinitis (the common cold) and is often associated with nasal polyps.

Complete loss of smell (anosmia) is unusual. It may follow a fracture of the cribriform plate where the olfactory neurons have been sheared off. It may also follow a viral infection. In both cases the loss of smell is usually permanent.

Malingerers often deny being able to smell gasoline fumes or ammonia. However these are sensed by the trigeminal nerve, which is unaffected by rhinitis.

Sneezing

This commonly occurs with allergic rhinitis and may be associated with itchy eyes and palate. Consider the possibility of coexistent asthma.

Pain

Pain from sinus disease is well localized. When the maxillary sinus is infected, the pain may radiate down into the upper teeth. If the sphenoid sinus is infected, the pain may present in the middle of the head. Characteristically, sinus pain is dull and persistent. The pain may last for several hours or days. It is aggravated by bending forward or straining (eg, nose blowing). Sinus pain is exacerbated by upper respiratory tract infections and occurs if there is pus within a sinus. Inadequate ventilation of a sinus may also cause pain; an example of this is the sinus headache that can occur with diving or flying. Not all facial pain is due to sinusitis—there are many other causes (eg, tension headaches, migraine, and dental pain).

Cosmetic Deformity

It is important to consider the cosmetic aspects of the nose. The patient may be unhappy about his or her appearance, but not volunteer the information spontaneously.

Other Points in the History

It is important to know if the patient has had any previous nasal surgery. A personal or family history of asthma, eczema, or hay fever suggests allergy; and bronchiectasis suggests possible ciliary dysfunction.

EXAMINATION

The External Nose and Face

The thickness, elasticity, and general condition of the skin are important when considering a patient for rhinopasty. Deviations or depressions of the nose are readily apparent. A finger passed over the dorsum of the nose allows the examiner to concentrate on defects in the nasal skeleton (Fig 11-2). A deviated septum is often apparent externally. Systemic disorders can affect the external appearance (eg, the saddling of Wegener's and the erythema and swelling of sarcoidosis). Gross nasal polyps (see Fig 16-3) may expand the nasal bones and in childhood a crease across the nose forms as a result of the allergic salute (Fig 11-3).

When testing the patency of a nasal airway, gently occlude one nostril with a finger (the thumb is ideal) (Fig 11-4). It is important not to deform the nasal airway under test by so doing.

Any objective swelling of the face suggests underlying infection or tumor. A patient with infective sinusitis may have tenderness under the supraorbital rim when this area is palpated.

Traditionally, the nasal cavity has been examined with a headlight or head mirror and a nasal speculum (Fig 11-5). Rigid endoscopes afford a much better view and with them the nasal cavity, its recesses and the postnasal space can be examined in great detail (Figs 11-6 through 11-9). An auriscope is a nonthreatening tool and is useful when examining small children (Fig 11-10).

If the nose is congested, the application of 10% cocaine spray causes vasoconstriction and thereby improves the view.

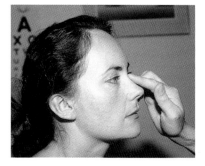

Fig 11-2 Gentle palpation of the dorsum of the nose detects underlying defects.

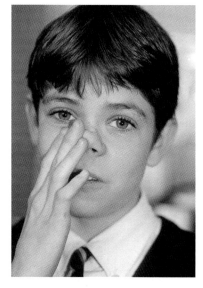

Fig 11-3 Children with severe allergic rhinitis frequently perform this allergic "salute."

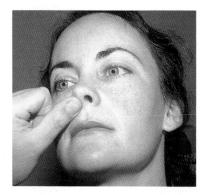

Fig 11-4 To test the patency of the nasal airway, one thumb gently occludes the nostril and the patient is asked to breathe in and out gently. The nostril being tested is not deformed.

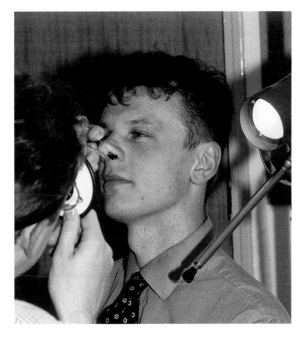

Fig 11-5 Examination conducted with a headlight and nasal speculum.

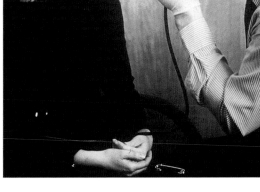

Fig 11-6 A patient undergoing nasal endoscopy.

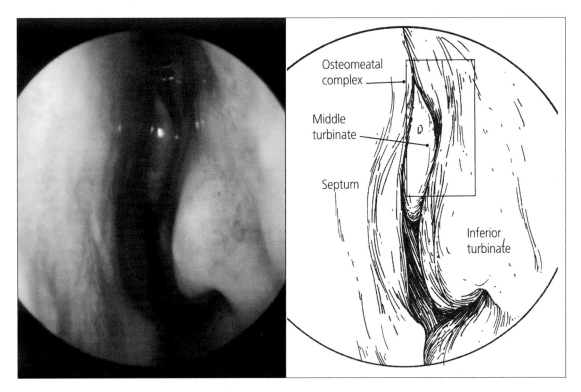

Fig 11-7 Endoscopic appearance of the left nostril in a normal nose. The septum is visible to the left, and the inferior turbinate and middle turbinates are also visible. Reprinted with permission from *American Family Physician.* 1998;58(3):708. Copyright 1998 by American Family Physician.

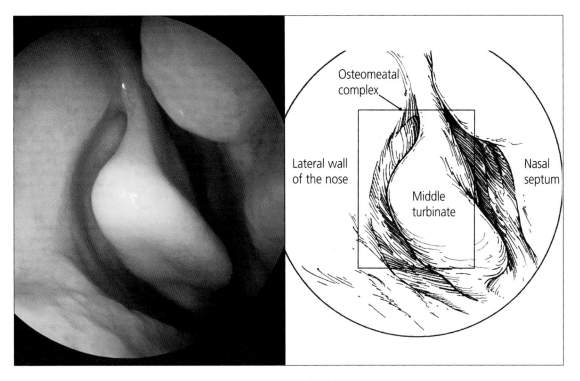

Fig 11-8 Endoscopic view of the middle turbinate, looking into the right nostril. The septum is to the right, with the lateral wall of the nose to the left. Reprinted with permission from *American Family Physician*. 1998;58(3):708. Copyright 1998 by American Family Physician.

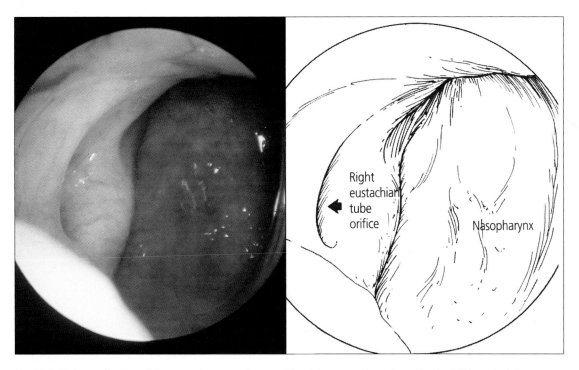

Fig 11-9 Endoscopic view of the normal postnasal space. The right eustachian tube orifice is visible to the left. Reprinted with permission from *American Family Physician*. 1998;58(3):708. Copyright American Family Physician.

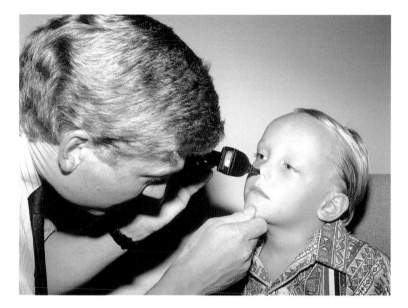

Fig 11-10 An otoscope is useful for nasal examination, especially when searching for a foreign body.

A normal mucous membrane is moist and pink. Abnormalities to look for include hypertrophic or occasionally atrophic mucosa and the presence of secretions and or crusting. Pus under the middle turbinate suggests sinus infection (Fig 11-11). Septal deformities, ulceration, granulation tissue, or any unilateral masses should be noted and require further investigation.

A hypertrophic turbinate (Fig 11-12) can be distinguished from a polyp (Fig 11-13) by gentle palpation with a probe. Polyps are pale gray, nontender, and mobile on palpation, whereas a turbinate is a

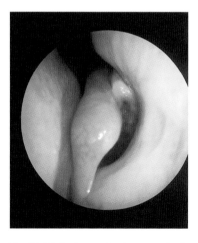

Fig 11-11 Endoscopic photograph of infective sinusitis.

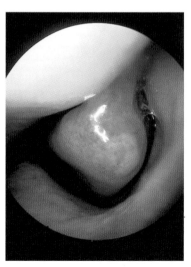

Fig 11-12 A hypertrophic inferior turbinate.

fixed structure with lots of nerve endings. Unilateral polyps should always be biopsied to exclude malignancy. Polyps are rare in children except when associated with cystic fibrosis.

The nose and sinuses should always be examined in conjuction with the rest of the head and neck. Remember that lymph drainage from the nose and sinuses goes to the neck.

Table 11-1 summarizes the main ingredients of history taking and nasal examination.

Table 11-1. Main Ingredients of History Taking and the Nasal Examination

Ear	Nose	Throat
History		
Earache, irritation	Obstruction	Hoarseness
Deafness	Rhinorrhoea/postnasal drip	Dysphagia
Discharge	Allergy/hay fever	Stridor
Tinnitus	Facial pain	Lump in the neck
Vertigo	Epistaxis	Sleep disturbance
	Sense of smell	
	Appearance	
Children: Speech/language		
Past History		
Barotrauma	Trauma	Cigarette smoking
Acoustic trauma	Medications	Alcohol
Head injury	Prescribed	
	Nonprescribed	
Ototoxics		
Family history	Previous surgery	
Previous ear surgery		
Examination		
Pinna	Shape	Mouth
Mastoid	Septum	(palates, gums, teeth, tonsils)
Ear canal	Turbinates	Neck
Eardrum (esp. attic)	Airway	Larynx refer to ENT
Tuning forks	Mucopus	
Conversational test	Facial tenderness	
Nystagmus	Facial sensation	
Facial nerve	Facial swelling	

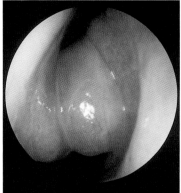

Fig 11-13 A nasal polyp. It is sometimes difficult to distinguish between hypertrophic turbinates and polyps. Turbinates are sensitie to palpation and contain bone that is attached to the lateral wall of the nose. A polyp is insensitive and is relatively mobile, swinging on a stalk that originates from an ethmoid air cell.

Key Points:

1. Unilateral nasal symptoms equal tumor or foreign body.

2. Bloodstained serosanguinous discharge equals tumor.

3. A unilateral nasal mass needs to be biopsied.

4. Clear watery rhinorrhoea can be due to leakage of cerebrospinal fluid.

5. Polyps are insensitive, mobile on palpation, and rare in children.

CHAPTER 12

Investigation of Nasal Function and Disease

RADIOLOGY

The sinuses are complex air-containing cavities within the skull. The sharp contrast between air and bone allows for good radiographic images.

Computerized Tomography (CT)

CT images bony structures well because of the high-density change between air and bone. A CT of the sinuses is usually taken in the coronal plane and 5-mm slices are used. Using the coronal plane reduces the radiation dose to the eye. If the coronal CT shows pathology in the posterior ethmoid cells, axial scans at the level of the optic nerve are recommended. CT is able to demonstrate the normal structures in fine detail as well as subtle or gross pathological changes (Figs 12-1 through 12-3). CT delineates nasal and sinus pathology and also acts as a route map for the endoscopic surgeon.

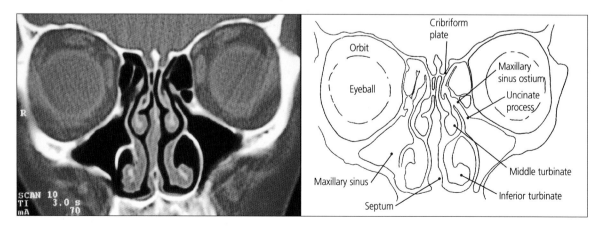

Fig 12-1 Coronal computed tomographic scan showing normal osteomeatal complex. Patient ostia are visible on both sides, and sinuses are well ventilated. Reprinted with permission from *American Family Physician.* 1998;58(3):708. Copyright 1998 by American Family Physician.

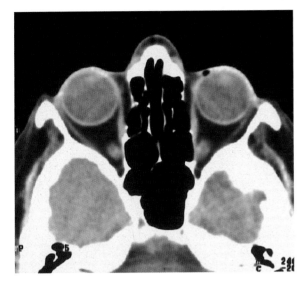

Fig 12-2 Normal axial CT of sinuses illustrating the close relationship of the optic nerve to posterior ethmoid sinuses. (Photograph courtesy of Dr. P. Anslow.)

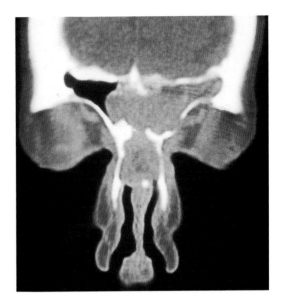

Fig 12-3 Coronal CT showing a mass in the ethmoid and frontal sinuses. A CT is good for showing bony detail.

Magnetic Resonance Imaging (MRI)

MRI demonstrates soft tissue abnormalities extremely well (Fig 12-4). Bone appears as a void. MRI is particularly useful for delineating tumor spread, although it may overestimate inflammatory disease.

Plain Radiographs

These are not recommended for routine use because they do not provide sufficient detail.

Angiography

Angiography is used to demonstrate the blood supply of vascular tumors (eg, angiofibromas). The relative importance of each feeding vessel can be demonstrated by angiography and embolization of feeding vessels can be performed to reduce tumor vascularity. Digital subtraction venous angiography allows noninvasive imaging of blood vessels.

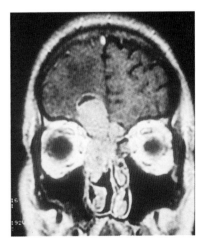

Fig 12-4 Sagittal MRI showing a nasal mass and its relationship to the frontal lobe. The MRI is good for illustrating the details of soft tissue.

Key Points:

1. CT is required before endoscopic sinus surgery.
2. CT identifies anatomical landmarks and variants and delineates pathology.
3. MRI is particularly useful for soft tissue masses (eg, tumors).
4. Mucosal thickening or fluid levels are not synonymous with infection.
5. Plain X rays are rarely useful and are not recommended.

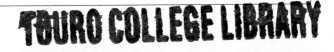

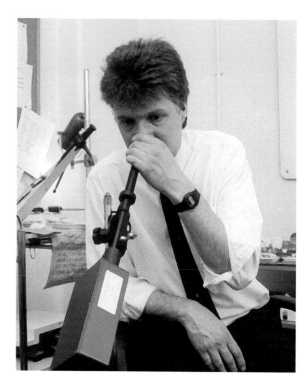

Fig 12-5 A patient using an acoustic rhinometer. A sound is pulsed into the nostril and the echoes are recorded. From this information an objective measurement of the spaces within the nasal cavity is made.

IMPEDANCE AND ACOUSTIC RHINOMANOMETRY

Impedance rhinometry measures the nasal airflow and pressure at the nostrils during respiration. These 2 parameters allow the nasal resistance to be calculated. Acoustic rhinometry works out the geography of the nasal cavity by pulsing a sound in through each nostril and recording the echoes (Fig 12-5). Both are objective measurements of nasal function, but with both methods it is difficult to easily obtain consistent results. Therefore, both methods remain research tools.

IMMUNOLOGICAL INVESTIGATION

Skin Tests

The common allergens that cause nasal allergy are wind-borne. Grass and tree pollen, animal proteins (house dust mite, dog hair, and cat fur), molds, and fungi are all implicated. The active component of these allergens can be isolated and mixed with glycerine to form a test solution.

Skin prick tests (Fig 12-6) are inexpensive, quick to perform, and a large number of allergens can be tested. Serious reactions to skin prick tests are exceedingly rare, provided that patients with a history of anaphylaxis are excluded and subcutaneous or

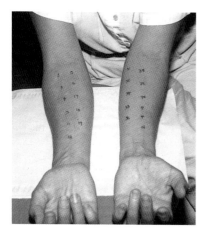

Fig 12-6 Skin test for allergy. Different antigens are numbered on the forearm and the reaction to antigen is compared to a histamine control.

intradermal injection is avoided. Skin prick tests provide useful supportive evidence (positive or negative) for a history suggestive of allergy. They provide a visual demonstration to the patient and they are essential when expensive allergy avoidance measures are being considered. Skin testing is a useful tool that helps patient education and allergy avoidance.

The Radio-allergo-sorbent Test (RAST)

In this test a sample of the patient's serum is taken and mixed with a known isolated allergen. If the patient is sensitive to the allergen, the IgE in the patient's serum binds with the antigen, and this is detected by adding radio-labeled anti-IgE. The RAST test is expensive but quantifies the allergic response and is particularly useful when skin tests cannot be undertaken.

Serum Immunoglobins

Chronic persistent sinusitis, especially in children, may result from hypogammaglobulinemia. The levels of IgG, IgA, and IgM can be measured. The importance of detecting these patients is that gammaglobulin deficiencies can be replaced. Various degrees of immune deficiency are common, so if in doubt send off some blood.

Other Tests

In patients with recurrent infections, it is worth checking the complete blood count, ESR, serum immunoglobins, urea, electrolytes, liver function tests, and blood and urine for sugar. There are specific antibody tests for certain diseases (eg, Wegener's granulomatosis).

INVESTIGATION OF MUCOCILIARY CLEARANCE

The Saccharin Test

This investigates movement of mucus within the nose and is a simple, cheap screening test (Fig 12-7). A small fragment of saccharin is placed on the anterior end of the inferior turbinate. The cilia sweep the mucus and saccharin back into the pharynx, at which point the patient tastes the saccharin. The time it takes for this to occur in a normal subject is about 10 minutes. If the test is negative, repeat it; if still abnormal, send the patient for brush biopsies to study ciliary function.

Brush Biopsy

A brush biopsy can be taken using a standard bronchoscopy brush. This is rubbed against the turbinates and the specimen is then mixed with saline. Under a phase contrast microscope, the

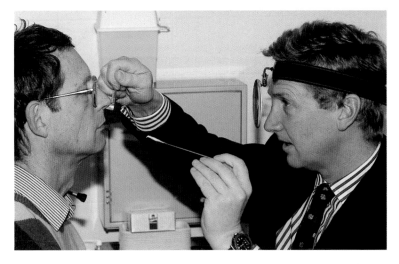

Fig 12-7 Mucociliary transport can be tested by placing a small amount of saccharin on the inferior turbinate. In the presence of active motile cilia clearance, the patient tastes the saccharin a few minutes later.

beat of normal ciliary action can be observed. This is an important test in the investigation of mucociliary disorders, but is available only in specialized centers. An early diagnosis of mucociliary disorders allows for regular physiotherapy to commence before permanent lung damage results.

BACTERIOLOGICAL INVESTIGATION

Routine nasal swabbing is of little diagnostic help because most of the organisms that cause sinus infection are also found in the normal nose (eg, *Streptococcus pneumoniae, Haemophilus influenzae, Streptococcus pyogenes*).

Infection that is resistant to antibiotics or infection in immunocompromised individuals should raise the suspicion of a fungal infection and a specimen should be sent for cytology.

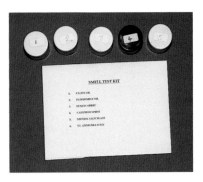

Fig 12-8 It is possible to test sense of smell with odors contained in bottles or on a smell strip. It is possible to obtain relevant smells for the particular region in which the patient lives.

Key Points:

1. A variety of investigations exist to detect allergy, immune deficiency, and mucociliary dysfunction in disorders of the nose and sinuses.

2. Skin tests, saccharin clearance, and immunoglobin screening are easy to do.

THE INVESTIGATION OF SMELL

It is possible to carry out a gross qualitative test of smell by using different scents (Fig 12-8). Some substances are detected by the trigeminal receptors and/or by the taste buds. Cinnamon is a scent that can only be detected by the olfactory neurons. It is clinically useful to know whether a smell is normal, reduced, or totally absent. Special smell testing strips are available. Ammonia can distinguish malingerers as it stimulates *the trigeminal nerve only.*

CHAPTER 13

Rhinosinusitis

Rhinitis affects 1 person in 6, and the incidence of seasonal rhinitis has increased fourfold over the last 20 years. Allergic rhinitis is the commonest immunological disorder and the commonest chronic disease in humans. This rise in the incidence of rhinitis may be due to pollutants which help initiate sensitization to inhaled allergens. Rhinitis and asthma frequently coexist and effective nasal treatment can improve pulmonary function.

Ciliated columnar epithelium extends throughout the sinuses and nasal passages which act together as one unit. Pathological changes in the nose are usually accompanied by similar findings in the sinuses, hence the term rhinosinusitis. With the exception of the occasional dental infection all sinusitis is caused by pathological changes in the nose, usually around the ostiomeatal complex. When using a classification (Table 13-1), it should be remembered

Table 13-1. The Classification of Rhinitis

Allergic	Infective	Other	Part of Systemic Disorder
Seasonal	Acute	Idiopathic	Primary defect in
Perennial	Chronic	NARES	mucus
Occupational		Drug-induced	Cystic fibrosis
		Beta blockers	Young's syndrome
		Oral contraceptive	Primary ciliary
		Aspirin	diskinesia
		NSAI	Kartagener's
		Topical	syndrome
		decongestants	Immunological
		Autonomic imbalance	SLE
		Atrophic	Rheumatoid arthritis
		Neoplastic	AIDS
			Antibody deficiency
			Granulomatous disease
			Wegener's,
			sarcoidosis
			Hormonal
			Hypothyroid
			Pregnancy

*Mechanical factors (eg, deviated septum, pneumatized middle turbinates) may partially obstruct the nose and sinus ostia and under these circumstances, mucosal inflammation may be more likely to cause rhinosinusitis.

that nasal problems are often multifactorial (eg, the swollen nasal mucosa caused by allergy may block the sinus ostia and thereby lead to infective rhinosinusitis).

ALLERGIC RHINITIS

Allergic rhinitis is common. The antigens that affect the nose are generally wind-borne (eg, grass and tree pollens), house dust mite, fungi, dog and cat dander. Allergic rhinitis may be seasonal, starting in early spring with tree pollen, followed by the grass pollen of midsummer, and finally the molds of autumn.

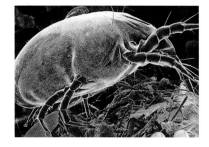

Fig 13-1 The house dust mite is the most common cause of perennial rhinitis.

The most common cause of perennial rhinitis is the house dust mite (Fig 13-1). The only way to completely escape this is to live in a mountain hut in Sweden (dry air, no carpets, etc). Paint solvents and other substances can cause occupational rhinitis, a subject that will assume more importance in the future.

The classic allergic reaction is the type 1 IgE-mediated reaction; immunoglobulin E (IgE) is produced from plasma cells, which in turn are regulated by T lymphocytes. IgE has a crystallizable fraction that binds to mast cells and an antigenbinding portion (Fab) that is free. When combined to an antigenic substance, the Fab portion triggers mast cell degranulation (Fig 13-2). The substances released include histamine, slow reacting substance of anaphylaxis (SRS-A), leukotrienes, and prostaglandins. These substances result in the production of mucosal edema and profuse nasal secretion.

Nonorganic substances can produce an inflammatory response. Nonspecific irritants, such as cigarette smoke and dust, cause the release of vasoactive substances, but the response is not IgE mediated. Sometimes nasal inflammation may be triggered by physical factors (temperature change), or dietary substances (eg, alcohol).

Occupational rhinitis occurs when the patient develops an allergy to substances at work (eg, latex, powders, paint vapors). A

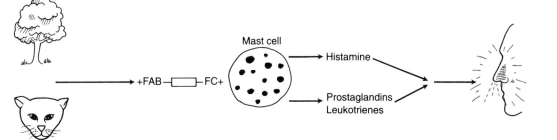

Fig 13-2 The IgE-mediated hypersensitivity reaction. The antigen binds with immunoglobin E, which then attaches to the mast cell. Mast cell degranulation causes the "hay fever" type symptoms.

careful history needs to be taken and the patient should improve when on vacation.

> **Key Points:**
>
> **1.** Seasonal allergic rhinitis occurs only when pollens are in the air (hay fever).
>
> **2.** Perennial rhinitis occurs all year round and can be caused by a myriad of substances, although house dust mite is high on the list.

INFECTIVE RHINOSINUSITIS

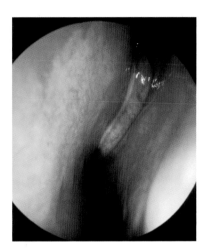

Fig 13-3 Infective rhinosinusitis with mucopus exuding out under the middle turbinate.

The best-known example of acute infective rhinosinusitis is the common cold. A large number of viruses have been implicated (influenza, para influenza, picorna, respiratory syncytial viruses, and adenoviruses). Infection is transmitted by droplet spread. The condition resolves or a secondary bacterial infection supervenes. *Haemophilus influenzae* and *Streptococcus pneumoniae* are the most common offenders.

Infective rhinosinusitis is characterized by a hypersecreting and hypertrophic nasal mucosa (Fig 13-3). When bacterial infection is present, the secretion becomes muco-purulent. Pus reduces the activity of cilia and this leads to stasis of secretions within the nose and sinuses.

Infection of the sinuses usually results from nasal infection, although, occasionally the maxillary sinus becomes infected directly from a dental abscess. The stages of sinus infection and predisposing factors are shown in (Fig 13-4). Infection of the nose and sinuses can lead to serious complications, which are discussed in Chapter 15 (p123-127).

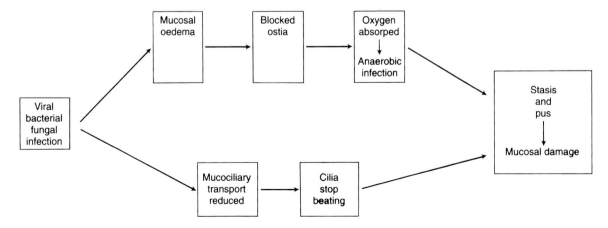

Fig 13-4 Stages in the development of sinus infection.

OTHER FORMS OF RHINITIS

These are rarer and include idiopathic (no obvious cause), NARES (nonallergic rhinitis with eosinophilia), drug-induced, autonomic imbalance, atrophic,and neoplastic.

Some of the drugs that can cause rhinitis are listed in Table 13-1.

Autonomic imbalance occurs when there is overstimulation by the parasympathetic nervous system. This produces a wet, swollen nose. There are two types of atrophic rhinitis:

1. *Rhinitis medicamentosa.* This is a condition brought about by the excessive use of vasoconstrictive sprays, which can be purchased without prescription. The spray constricts the blood vessels in the nose and rapidly relieves nasal blockage. A rebound hyperemia occurs after 2 to 3 hours so that more spray is required to produce relief. A vicious cycle is entered with some individuals becoming dependent on the spray. Topical vasoconstrictor nasal sprays should not be used for more than a few weeks.

2. *Atrophic rhinitis not induced by medication.* This is an uncommon condition associated with excessive crusting and dryness in the nose. The nostrils become widely patent and the nose crusts and smells horribly. It may follow radical nasal surgery in which most of the nasal "furniture" has been removed. It may occasionally have an infective cause because *Klebsiella* is often cultured in this condition.

RHINITIS ASSOCIATED WITH PART OF A SYSTEMIC DISORDER

Primary Defect in the Mucus

Cystic fibrosis may present with nasal polyps in a person under the age of 20, and in Young's syndrome the patient presents with recurrent rhiniosinusitis that does not respond to conventional treatment. Mucous transport is impaired so that the saccharin transit is delayed or does not occur (p102).

Primary Ciliary Dyskinesia

Nasal cilia beat in a coordinated manner about 14 times a second so that a thin blanket of mucus moves throughout the nasal cavity and sinuses. In Kartagener's syndrome the cilia beat in a discoordinated manner so the mucociliary transport system fails. It is important to diagnose this condition early because chest physiotherapy and selective use of antibiotics may prevent bronchiectasis.

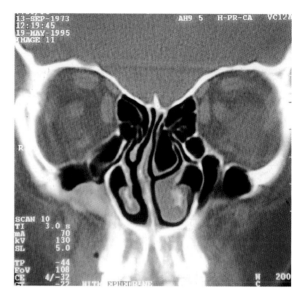

Fig 13-5 Coronal CT showing a pneumatized middle turbinate (concha bullosa) and a deviated septum.

MECHANICAL FACTORS

Anatomical obstruction can result from a deviated septum or enlarged turbinate (Fig 13-5). In the presence of severe obstruction mucosal inflammation is more likely to lead to severe rhinosinusitis.

MEDICAL TREATMENT OF RHINOSINUSITIS

The first principle is to treat the underlying cause.

Allergen Avoidance

If there is a strong history of allergy, this can be investigated with skin tests and the patient can then be advised how best to avoid the antigens.

House Dust Mite Avoidance

The major allergen in house dust mite feces has now been identified as Der pI. House dust mites are found in mattresses, pillows, duvets, carpets,and soft furnishing including cuddly toys! Mites propogate fast in a warm, well-insulated house. Gortex mattress covers, washing the bedclothes at 60°C, replacing carpets with wood floors, and putting the teddy bear in the freezer have been shown to reduce the mite count. Some of these measures are expensive and are worth doing only if the subject has been shown to be allergic to mite on skin testing.

Seasonal Rhinitis (Hay Fever)

Total avoidance of pollens is not possible but simple measures can reduce exposure (eg, keeping windows shut on a summer evening, pollen filters in the car, and wearing sunglasses). Alternatively, advise the patient to take a vacation near the sea during the peak pollen season.

Avoiding Animal Allergens

This can be a tricky subject. The major cat allergen (Fel dI) is a salivary protein that is preened onto the fur at regular intervals. Cat allergen stays in the air for many months. Ideally families with atopic members should be advised against having furry animals in the home. However, once a family has become attached to a pet, the best advice may be to ban the animal from the bedrooms and main living area. It has been shown that washing the cat once a week reduces the antigen levels, but this presents a formidable challenge.

Immunotherapy or Desensitization

It is occasionally possible to desensitize a patient by injecting increasing concentrations of the allergen that is responsible for the allergy. This method is only useful in carefully selected individuals who have an allergy that is caused by a specific antigen that has been identified with skin prick testing or RAST. An ideal patient for desensitization would have an allergy to one type of grass pollen only. Patients with multiple allergies should be excluded. Patients with asthma should also be excluded because there is a risk of anaphylaxis. The mechanism of immunotherapy is largely unknown, although "tolerance" of T cells is involved. It is recommended that immunotherapy only be given where there are facilities for full resuscitation. The patient should be closely observed for at least 30 minutes after treatment.

PHARMACOLOGICAL TREATMENT OF RHINOSINUSITIS

Infective rhinosinusitis should initially be treated with antibiotics and vasoconstrictor nose drops. Medical treatment for chronic rhinosinusitis should be combined with allergy avoidance measures. The mainstay of treatment for allergic rhinitosinusitis is topical corticosteroids and antihistamines, with systemic corticosteroids held in reserve for severe cases. Mast cell stablilizers (cromoglycate) and topical anticholinergic sprays also have a role. Medical treatment for rhinitis is highly effective if the patient complies.

Topical Steroids and Cromoglycate

Topical steroid *sprays* act in a prophylactic manner and need to be taken on a daily basis. They are not associated with systemic side effects. Topical steroid *drops* are more potent and are best used at the start of treatment to establish control before swapping to a spray. Topical corticosteroids act in a number of different ways but can generally be considered to have an antiinflammatory action. For maximal effect in seasonal rhinitis, the spray should be commenced before the season and should be used throughout the season. Effective treatment is all about compliance and patient education. The most common reason for treatment failure with topical steroids is simply that the patient has not taken the spray correctly.

Topical sodium cromoglycate represents an alternative anti-inflammatory agent and is particularly useful in children. A disadvantage is that it needs to be taken 4 times a day, which makes compliance difficult.

Systemic Steroids

Courses of oral corticosteroids may be needed for severe symptoms (eg, when nasal blockage is so bad that access for a topical spray is impossible). A nose full of polyps will also respond in the short term to oral steroids. A minimum effective dose would be 20 mg of prednisilone daily for 5 days. The patient should be aware that systemic steroids have side effects and adverse reactions.

Antihistamines

Antihistamines are particularly effective for symptoms of sneezing, itching, and watery rhinorrhea, but have little effect on nasal blockage. They do have the advantage of being effective for the eye, palatal, and throat symptoms associated with allergy. The newer antihistamines produce very little sedation and psychomotor impairment. They can be used in combination with topical corticosteroids.

Anticholinergic

Ipratropium bromide is available as a nasal spray and it blocks the parasympathetic nervous system. Its main use is controlling profuse watery rhinorrhea.

Key Points:

1. Drug treatment should be combined with allergy avoidance.

2. The majority of patients on topical treatment do not take it correctly.

Antibiotics

The initial treatment of an acute infective rhinosinusitis includes appropriate antibiotics combined with a vasoconstrictor spray. An antibiotic that covers anaerobic bacteria should be chosen. The rationale for the vasoconstrictor spray is that it reduces mucosal swelling and can open up the sinus ostia.

Surgical Treatment

The surgical treatments available for all forms of rhinosinusitis are discussed in the next chapter.

CHAPTER 14

Surgical Treatment for Patients With Sinus and Nasal Pathology

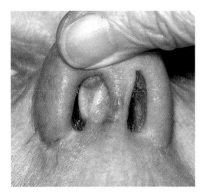

Fig 14-1 The caudal end of the septum is displaced into this man's right nostril. Gentle elevation of the columella reveals the deformity.

SEPTAL AND TURBINATE SURGERY

Etiology

Septal deviation may result from genetic factors, birth trauma, or injury later in life. The deviation may be either in the cartilaginous or bony components or both.

Clinical Features

The usual symptom is of nasal obstruction. This is often unilateral. However, the obstruction may involve both nostrils due to the effects of the nasal cycle superimposed on a deviated septum. If the nose is deviated (Fig 14-1), as is commonly the case, it may be cosmetically unacceptable. A patient with a deviated septum is predisposed to sinusitis and the altered airflow may also lead to a dry mucosa, which subsequently bleeds.

Patients with septal deformity vary greatly in terms of their symptoms. Some with a grossly deviated septum do not have any problems. Others feel that the nose is blocked when there is only minimal septal deviation present.

An assessment of the degree of nasal obstruction can be made clinically (p94).

Treatment

A slight septal deviation will not need treatment—remember that few septums are strictly in the midline!

If there is cosmetic deformity or nasal obstruction, surgical treatment is recommended. The operation to correct a deviated septum is called a septoplasty. The attachments of the quadrilateral cartilage are dissected free and then the cartilage is repositioned in the midline.

The complications of septal surgery include septal perforation, collapse of the nasal dorsum, and adhesions between the septum and the lateral wall of the nose.

Turbinate Surgery

Nasal obstruction can be caused by an excessively pneumatized middle turbinate and this anatomical variation is called a concha bullosa (see Fig 13-5). In the presence of a unilateral concha bullosa, the septum is usually deviated to the opposite side. Mechanical obstruction caused by a concha bullosa can be cured by endoscopic resection of part of the bone, often combined with a septoplasty.

Mucosal hypertrophy of the inferior turbinates usually responds to medical treatment but in persistent cases the obstruction can be relieved by surgery.

A variety of surgical procedures are available to reduce the bulk of the swollen turbinates (cryosurgery, submucous diathermy, cautery, and trimming of the turbinates). All of these methods may lead to an improved nasal airway and better access for topical medical treatment.

FUNCTIONAL ENDOSCOPIC SINUS SURGERY (FESS)

Functional Endoscopic Sinus Surgery (FESS) is a minimally invasive technique, the aim of which is to restore sinus ventilation and normal function. Fiberoptic telescopes are used for diagnosis and for the surgical technique. These endoscopes provide a quality view of the recesses within the nasal cavity. Computerized tomography (CT) identifies the anatomy and diseased areas.

FESS should be reserved for patients in whom medical treatment has failed. The patients who do best with FESS are those with recurrent acute or chronic infective sinusitis. These patients can expect an 80% to 90% improvement in their symptoms. FESS is suitable for outpatient surgery and patients usually experience minimal discomfort. External scars are avoided. The complication rate with FESS is lower than with "conventional" nonendoscopic sinus surgery. FESS requires special training.

Fiberoptic endoscopes have made it possible to examine the nose thoroughly from the anterior nares to the postnasal space using local anesthetic in the office (see Figs 11-8, 11-9, and 11-10). The specific features that need to be assessed on examination are the middle turbinate and middle meatus (ostiomeatal complex), anatomical obstruction, mucopus, and/or nasal polyps (Figs 14-2 and 14-3).

CT scanning identifies the anatomical relationships of the key structures (orbital contents, optic nerve, and carotid artery) to the diseased areas, a process that is vital for surgical planning. CT defines the extent of disease in any individual sinus, and also any underlying anatomical variants that may predispose an individual to sinusitis (Figs 14-4 through 14-6).

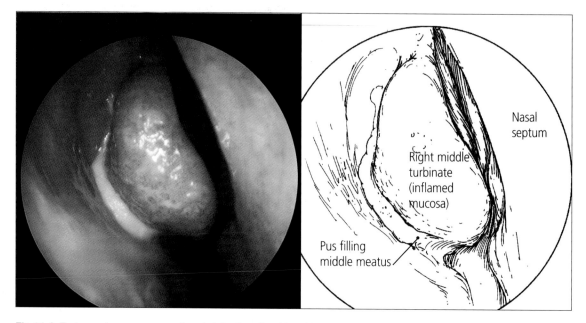

Fig 14-2 Endoscopic appearance of acute infective sinusitis, with pus exuding from under the right middle turbinate and down into the middle meatus. Reprinted with permission from *American Family Physician*. 1998;58(3):709. Copyright 1998 by American Family Physician.

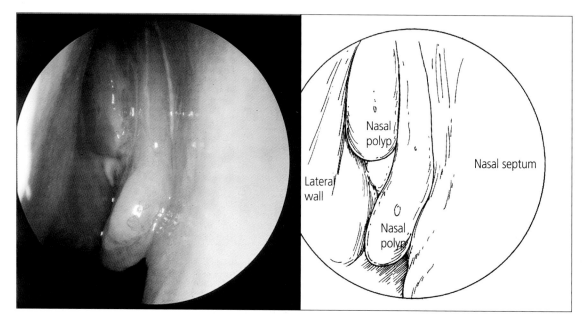

Fig 14-3 Nasal polyps in the left nostril, blocking the ostiomeatal complex. Reprinted with permission from *American Family Physician*. 1998;58(3):709. Copyright 1998 by American Family Physician.

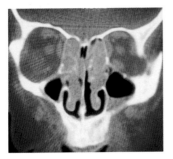

Fig 14-4 Coronal computed tomographic scan showing ethmoidal polyps. Ethmoid opacity is total as a result of nasal polyps, with a secondary fluid level in the maxillary antrum. Reprinted with permission from *American Family Physician.* 1998;58(3):710. Copyright 1998 by American Family Physician.

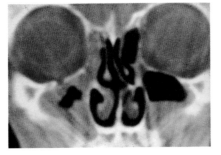

Fig 14-5 Coronal computed tomographic scan showing rhinosinusitis with a blocked ostiomeatal complex and secondary infection in the maxillary sinuses. Reprinted with permission from *American Family Physician.* 1998;58(3):77. Copyright 1998 by American Family Physician.

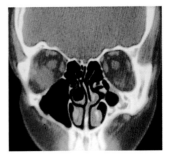

Fig 14-6 computed tomographic scan showing developed right middle turbinate (concha bullosa) and a deviated nasal septum. Reprinted with permission from *American Family Physician.* 1998;58(3):711. Copyright 1998 by American Family Physician.

The aim of FESS is to return the mucociliary drainage of the sinuses to normal function.

The rationale behind FESS is that localized pathology in the ostiomeatal complex blocks the ostia and leads to inflammation in the dependent sinuses. The surgical interventions of FESS are designed to remove the ostiomeatal blockage and restore normal sinus ventilation and muco-ciliary function (Fig 14-7).

The Surgical Techniques for FESS

The nose is prepared with a vasoconstrictor (eg, cocaine or ephedrine). The middle turbinate is identified. This is the most important landmark for the whole procedure. On the lateral wall of the nose at the level of the anterior end of the middle turbinate lies the uncinate process. This is removed (Fig 14-8), exposing the ethmoid bulla and the opening called the hiatus semiluminaris into which the frontal and maxillary sinuses drain.

The anterior ethmoid cells are then opened, allowing better ventilation but leaving the bone covered with mucosa. Following this, the maxillary ostium is inspected. If obstructed, it can be opened by performing a middle meatal antrostomy (Fig 14-9). This minimal surgery will often be sufficient to greatly improve the function of the ostiomeatal complex and therefore provide better ventilation of the maxillary, ethmoid, and frontal sinuses.

The results after FESS are good with most papers reporting an 80% to 90% success rate.

The complication rate of FESS is lower than the older "open" techniques. The most catastrophic and most mentioned complication of

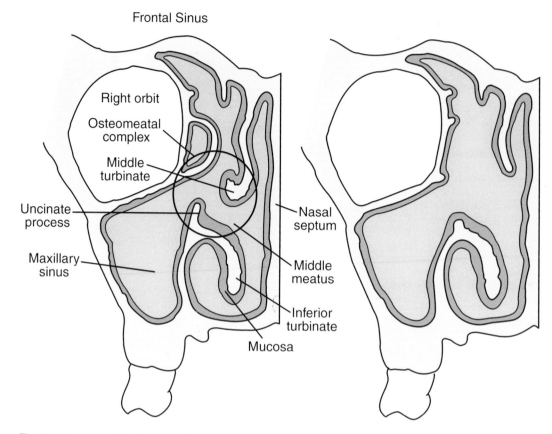

Fig 14-7 Anatomy of the sinuses. Left, narrowing in the circled region (middle meatus, middle turbinate, uncinate process) may precipitate sinusitis. Right, after functional endoscopic sinus surgery, the osteomeatal area is open. Reprinted with permission from *American Family Physician.* 1998;58(3):709. Copyright 1998 by American Family Physician.

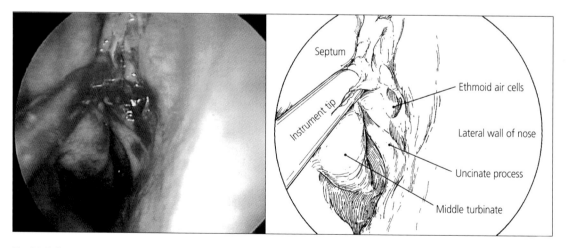

Fig 14-8 Surgical removal of the uncinate process. Reprinted with permission from *American Family Physician.* 1998;58(3):715. Copyright 1998 by American Family Physician.

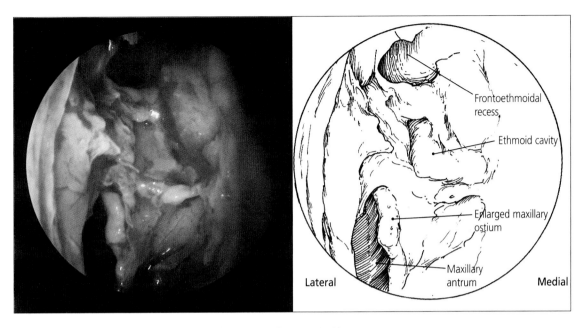

Frontoethmoidal recess

Ethmoid cavity

Enlarged maxillary ostium

Maxillary antrum

Lateral   Medial

Fig 14-9 A middle meatal antrostomy in the right nostril. Reprinted with permission from *American Family Physician.* 1998;58(3):715. Copyright 1998 by American Family Physician.

FESS is blindness due to damage to the optic nerve. However, the evidence is that the frequency of this complication is extremely low. Cerebrospinal leak is the single most common complication, occurring in about 0.2% of cases. The leak is usually recognized at the time of surgery and can be easily repaired, but it should be suspected if there is a clear nasal discharge postoperatively. Absolute confirmation of CSF can be obtained by sending off a sample to see if it contains Beta 2 transferrin.

Other less serious but equally rare complications include orbital hematoma (Fig 14-10) and nasal lacrimal duct stenosis.

Extended Uses of FESS

Endoscopic Dacryocystorhinostomy (DCR)

This procedure is usually performed by an otolaryngologist and an ophthalmic surgeon working together. It can be done in an office under local anesthesia. The blockage within the tear duct is confirmed with a contrast dacrocystogram (Fig 14-11). The ophthalmic surgeon dilates the duct and passes a fine, flexible fiberoptic light lead down the duct so that the endoscopic surgeon can identify the light in the lateral wall of the nose, usually just in front of the middle turbinate. The endoscopist uses a microdrill or laser to remove the bone overlying the duct. Stents are then inserted

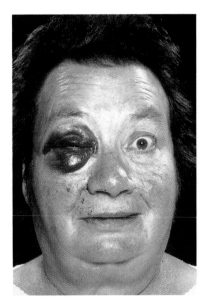

Fig 14-10 Orbital hematoma—a rare complication of FESS. (Photograph provided courtesy of Mr. R. Slack.)

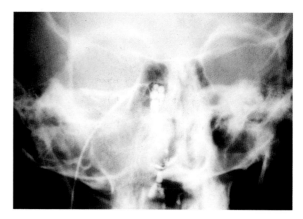

Fig 14-11 A contrast dacryocystogram showing blockage of the tear duct in the lateral wall of the nose.

and left in place for 6 weeks. The success rate is equal to external DCR (80-90%) and an external incision is avoided.

Endoscopic Orbital Decompression

The indications for this procedure are optic neuropathy and the problems associated with the exopthalmos of thyroid eye disease (Figs 14-12 through 14-14). Endoscopic decompression of the orbit is achieved by fully exenterating the ethmoid air cells and then removing the thin bone (lamina papyracea) that forms the medial wall of the orbit.

Access to Areas That Are Difficult to Reach

The endoscope allows the surgeon to access areas that are difficult to view with conventional techniques (eg, the sphenoid

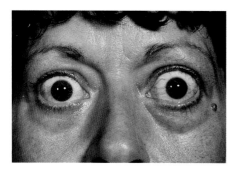

Fig 14-12 Proptosis of thyroid eye disease causes a cosmetic deformity and the patient frequently complains of a heavy pressure feeling in and around the eyes.

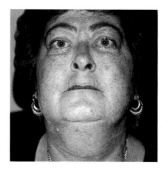

Fig 14-13 The inflammation of thyroid eye disease limits movement of the globe and this patient has to tip her head backwards in order to see straight ahead.

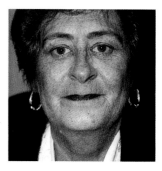

Fig 14-14 Same patient after endoscopic orbital decompression.

sinus). It is possible to drain most frontal, ethmoidal, or sphenoidal mucoceles (Fig 14-15). Small pituitary surgery tumors can also be removed endoscopically.

Tumor Diagnosis and Monitoring

The endoscopes provide a brilliant view of the hidden recesses of the nasal cavity and the sinuses. With these tools, the surgeon is able to see most rhinological tumors and biopsy them directly. Following definitive treatment, the endoscopes are extremely useful for checking the nose to exclude recurrence.

CSF Leak Repair

CSF leaks can occur from the cribriform plate region and the sphenoid. These areas are accessible to the surgeon with an endoscope and most CSF leaks can now be repaired endoscopically, avoiding craniotomy (Figs 14-16 and 14-17).

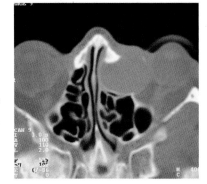

Fig 14-15 CT scan of an ethmoidal mucocele, which was subsequently drained using an endoscopic approach.

Key Points:

1. FESS is best reserved for patients with persistent or recurrent rhinosinusitis despite medical treatment.

2. FESS is a minimally invasive technique that attempts to restore normal function by correcting problems within the nose.

3. The indications for "conventional" sinus surgery are now few.

4. Endoscopic techniques are now used for tear duct surgery, orbital decompression, and in the management of malignant disease.

Sinus Washouts

This is now rarely done as an isolated procedure but is often performed during endoscopic sinus surgery. The maxillary sinus can be washed out as part of the treatment of acute or chronic sinusitis (Fig 14-18). Infected returns are sent for culture and sensitivity.

Radical Antrostomy or Caldwell-Luc Operation

The advent of endoscopic sinus surgery has all but eliminated the need for this procedure in chronic sinusitis. The operation (Fig 14-19) involves removal of part of the anterior wall of the maxillary sinus to gain entry to it. It was thought that at some point the sinus lining became irreversibly damaged and was best removed. The radical antrostomy operation was used to do this. Endoscopic surgery to restore sinus ventilation has shown that even a severely infected sinus lining can usually recover when it is exposed to fresh air.

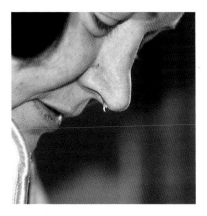

Fig 14-16 Patient presenting with a spontaneous CSF leak confirmed by the presence of Beta 2 transferrin.

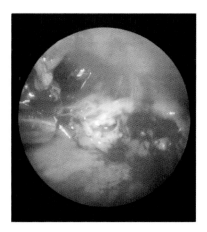

Fig 14-17 a. Endoscopic photograph of patient shown in Fig 14-16, showing a hole in the cribriform plate through which CSF was pouring. **b.** Coronal CT scan of same patient with a CSF leak. Fluid levels can be seen in the right ethmoid and right maxillary sinus. **c.** The 3-D CT reconstruction of the cribriform plate region made preoperatively in an attempt to identify the site of the leak.

Fig 14-17a

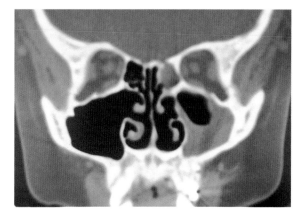

Fig 14-17b

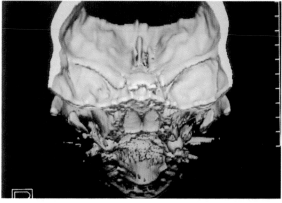

Fig 14-17c

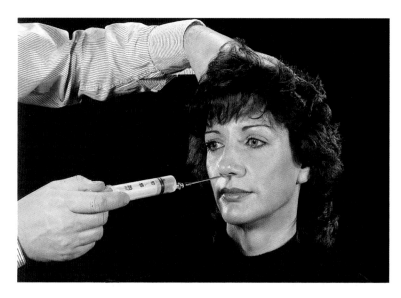

Fig 14-18 Sinus washout under local anesthesia. Now rarely performed.

The radical antrostomy approach is still used occasionally for access to the maxillary sinus and its relations (eg, to lift a fractured orbital floor).

External Ethmoidectomy

This operation (Fig 14-20) is used for decompressing the orbit when acute ethmoiditis threatens vision. Under these circumstances, endoscopic techniques are difficult because the inflamed tissues bleed excessively.

Frontal Sinus Trephine

This procedure (Fig 14-21) is indicated when the frontoethmoidal recess remains blocked despite conservative treatment. Only a small skin incision is required and a drill is used to trephine the bone. Through this hole pus can be drained and a telescope can be inserted. This allows endoscopic surgeons to work from above and below to open up the frontoethmoidal recess if it is blocked off (Fig 14-22).

Midfacial Degloving

This approach provides excellent access to the middle third of the face and external incisions are avoided (Figs 14-23 and 14-24). The approach is used for the resection of large benign tumors (eg,

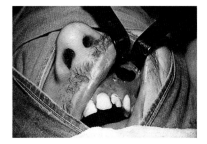

Fig 14-19 The radical antrostomy or Caldwell-Luc operation used to be performed for chronic sinusitis. It is now mainly used as an approach for repairing orbital floor fractures.

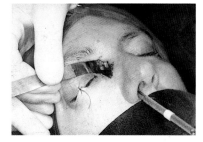

Fig 14-20 The external ethnoidectomy operation is used for decompressing the orbit to relieve pressure caused by acute ethmoid infection.

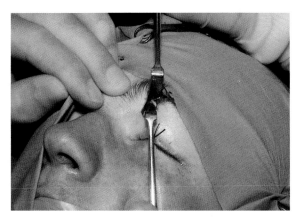

Fig 14-21 Frontal sinus trephine.

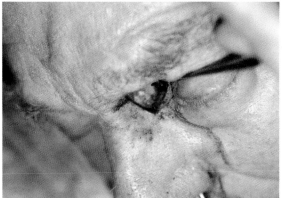

Fig 14-22 Disease of the frontal sinus is difficult to treat. This photograph illustrates a combined approach. The endoscopic surgeon has approached from below and the light of the endoscope can be seen shining into the frontal sinus after the latter has been opened by a small incision. Two surgeons are able to work from above and below in order to reestablish frontal sinus ventilation. (Photograph provided courtesy of Mr. R. Corbridge.)

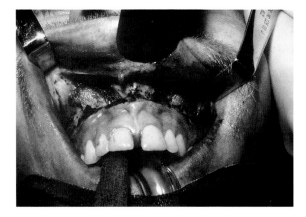

Fig 14-23 The midfacial degloving approach leaves no external scars and gives good access to the middle third of the face. (Photograph provided courtesy of Mr. R. Slack.)

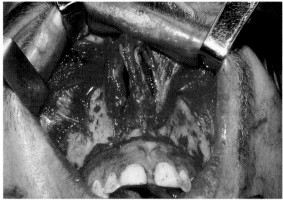

Fig 14-24 The midfacial degloving approach may be used for tumor resection or repair of fractures. (Photograph provided courtesy of Mr. R. Slack.)

juvenile angiofibroma; see p. 154, Fig 20-3) and selected malignant tumors (eg, carcinoma of the maxilla; see p. 156, Fig 20-7).

Craniofacial Resection

The craniofacial approach is used to resect malignant tumors of the sinuses. The ethmoid sinuses and attached dura can be removed *en bloc* and orbital exenteration and maxillectomy can be performed as well, if required.

The Complications of Rhinosinusitis

The complications of sinusitis can be serious and life-threatening. The most common causes of intracranial sepsis are chronic sinus disease and chronic ear disease.

ORBITAL COMPLICATIONS

These most frequently follow ethmoidal and frontal sinusitis. Pus under pressure may breach the thin lamina papyracea (Figs 15-1 through 15-4) that forms the medial wall of the orbit. Infection can then spread to the orbital contents via veins or by breaching the periostium. Orbital cellulitis can occur within a few hours of the onset of symptoms (Table 15-1). Acute ethmoiditis is relatively common in childhood. If a child presents with a proptosed red eye, it is likely to be acute ethmoiditis and not simply an eye infection.

Treatment involves urgent hospital admission, intravenous antibiotics, and monitoring of visual acuity. An urgent CT scan is always helpful and will delineate if the infection lies anterior

Table 15–1. Presentation of Orbital Complications of Acute Sinusitis

Swollen eyelids and proptosis
Restricted eye movements
Reduction of visual acuity

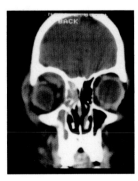

Fig 15-1 Coronal CT showing acute ethmoiditis. The lamina papyracea has been breached and there is pus in the orbit. (Photograph courtesy of Mr. C Milford.)

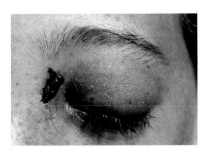

Fig 15-2 The patient whose CT is shown in Fig 15-1 with pus discharging out through a tract at the medial camphus. (Photo courtesy of Mr. C Milford.)

CHAPTER 15

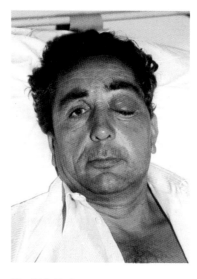

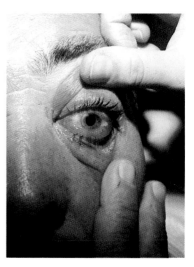

Fig 15-3 Patient with acute ethmoiditis.

Fig 15-4 It is important to examine the eye to check the visual acuity.

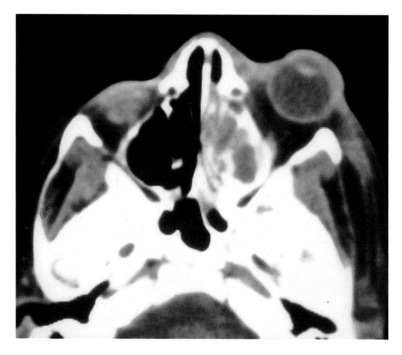

Fig 15-5 An axial CT scan demonstrating infective ethmoiditis.

(preseptal) or posterior in the ethmoids (postseptal) (Fig 15-5). The septum is a reflection of periosteum into the tarsal plate. CT will also show the extent of infection—whether, for example, the orbital periosteum has been breached. If there is deterioration of visual acuity, the orbital contents need to be decompressed.

Key Points:

1. The most common causes of intracranial sepsis are chronic sinus disease and chronic ear disease. Anaerobic organisms are often involved.

2. Acute ethmoiditis can cause loss of vision. Early, intensive antibiotic therapy in hospital is necessary.

OSTEOMYELITIS

Osteomyelitis of the frontal bone spreads from infection within the frontal sinuses. The patient in Figures 15-6 and 15-7 has a "Potts Puffy tumor": pus has tracked up from the frontal sinus through diploic bone. In young patients the anterior bony wall of the maxillary antrum may be diploic and osteomyelitis can follow a maxillary sinusitis.

INTRACRANIAL COMPLICATIONS

Infection of the ethmoid or frontal sinuses may spread to the cranial cavity via a bony defect, emissary veins, or via a thrombosed vessel (eg, lateral sinus). *Any combination of meningitis, extradural, subdual, or intracerebral abscess is possible.* Usually a history of preceding sinusitis can be obtained from the patient or relatives.

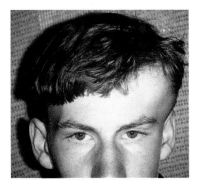

Fig 15-6 A patient with a Pott's puffy tumor.

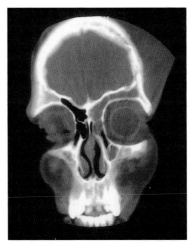

Fig 15-7 The CT scan of the patient shown in Fig 15-6. Pus has tracked up from the frontal sinus through the diploic bone until it presents at a suture line.

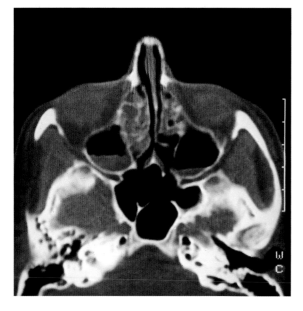

Fig 15-8 CT scan showing pansinusitis.

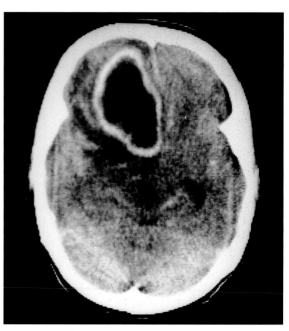

Fig 15-9 Sinusitis has led to a frontal lobe abscess. It is important to think of this complication if a diagnosis is to be made. This particular patient simply appeared somewhat vague with a headache.

Subdural Abscess

This can be difficult to diagnose. A typical history is of a young adolescent male who has sustained sinus trauma. It may not be diagnosed until the patient is unconscious because the signs are subtle initially. They include headache, pyrexia, and fits, and there may be localized neurological signs. Even with a high-resolution CT scan, it can be difficult to pick up such a collection of pus.

Intracerebral Abscess (Figs 15-8 and 15-9)

The frontal lobe is a relatively "silent" area and it is usually this lobe that is affected. Initially the patient may not appear ill, but as the abscess forms, drowsiness and a reduced level of consciousness may occur. Fits and papilloedema may be present. Treatment requires neurosurgical consultation and involves an intensive antibiotic regimen and repeated aspiration and drainage of the abscess.

Cavernous Sinus Thrombosis (Fig 15-10)

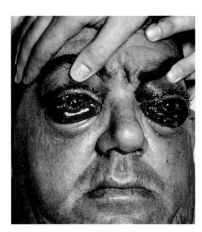

Fig 15-10 Cavernous sinus thrombosis—a rare and usually fatal complication of sinusitis.

Part of the venous drainage of the nose and sinuses is to the cavernous sinus. Thankfully, cavernous sinus thrombosis is rare, but when it does occur it follows infection in the orbit, face, nose, or sinuses. Illness may appear quickly with a sharp rise in temperature, proptosis, and pain in the eyes. There is swelling of the conjunctiva and eyelids and ophthalmoplegia develops. This condition has a high mortality.

Key Points:

1. The most common cause of intracranial sepsis is an infected sinus or an infected ear.

2. Any combination of meningitis, extradural, subdural, or intracerebral abscess may follow sinus infection.

3. The onset of headache, photophobia, drowsiness, rigors, or personality change in a patient with sinus disease should always raise the possibility of intracranial suppuration.

4. A normal CT scan does not exclude intracranial suppuration, especially early in the course of the infection.

CHAPTER 16

Two Entities: Nasal Polyps and Septal Perforations

NASAL POLYPS

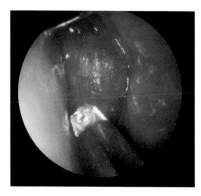

Fig 16-1 Various power tools now available to remove nasal polyps with minimal trauma.

Nasal polyps are considered as a separate entity because their etiology is not known. They are pale gray sacks of mucosa that hang down into the nasal cavity (Fig 16-1).

Each polyp usually forms in an ethmoidal air cell, and the polyp is the grossly swollen lining of the sinus. Although the disease process mainly affects the ethmoids, polypoid change can occur elsewhere in the nose and other sinuses.

The etiology of nasal polyps is not fully understood. There is no evidence that infection causes nasal polyps, although infective sinusitis may result from polyps blocking the sinus ostia. An allergic etiology has been proposed because 90% of polyps contain an increased number of eosinophils. Eosinophils, however, are not specific for allergy and positive skin tests are no more common in patients with nasal polyps than in controls.

Nasal polyps can occur at any age but are uncommon in childhood. Nasal polyps are more common in men although the sex incidence is equal in patients who also have asthma. Most nasal polyps are bilateral. *Beware of the unilateral polyp; it always needs to be biopsied as it may be an inverting papilloma or a carcinoma.*

A consistent finding is that the fluid inside a polyp contains a high level of histamine (100 to 1000 times that of serum). This implies that mast cell degranulation occurs. The products of mast cell release may not be cleared from the ethmoid mucosa as rapidly as from other tissues because of the relatively poor blood supply. In addition to allergy, several other factors can cause mast cell degranulation (eg, temperature change, various drugs, and complement factors).

There is a close link with asthma, so that 50% of patients presenting with nasal polyps will already have or will develop asthma. Treating the nasal polyps reduces the nasal resistance and usually improves the chest symptoms. In 8% of patients with nasal polyps, there is a triad consisting of nasal polyps, asthma, and aspirin sensitivity (ASA or Sempter's triad). Patients with this triad generally have a miserable time (Figs 16-2 and 16-3). They may respond to a salicylate-free diet, although this is a difficult diet to comply with.

Nasal polyposis is a chronic condition with a high incidence of recurrence, whichever treatment regime is pursued.

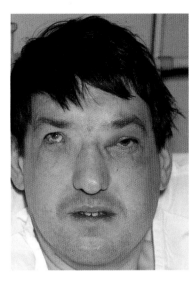

Fig 16-2

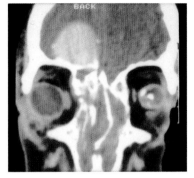

Fig 16-3

Fig 16-2 A patient with ASA triad (asthma, polyps, and Aspirin sensitivity). This patient was born blind in one eye and the nasal polyps were so prolific they were pushing his good eye out of its socket.

Fig 16-3 A CT scan of the same patient showing gross polyposis.

Clinical Features

The most common symptoms are nasal obstruction, rhinorrhea and postnasal drip (Figs 16-4 and 16-5). The discharge may be clear, yellow, or green depending on the degree of eosinophilia or infection.

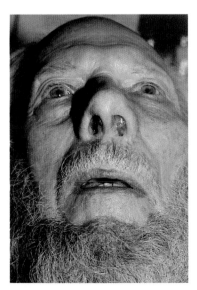

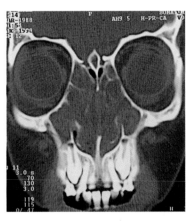

Fig 16-5 CT scan of the same patient showing "total whiteout" (opacity throughout the sinuses).

Fig 16-4 Patient with polyps totally blocking his nose. Note that simple nasal polyps are bilateral.

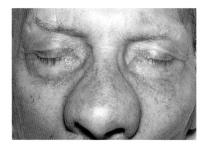

Fig 16-6 A "frog face" caused by nasal polyps splaying the nasal bones.

Sneezing and reduction in the sense of smell are frequent but pain is unusual unless the sinuses are secondarily infected. Bleeding or a serosanguinous discharge is unusual and, if present, a carcinoma should be suspected.

On examination, the voice is hyponasal, as if the person has a permanent cold. Polyps are bilateral and appear as pale, glistening gray sacks hanging down into the nose. It is possible to distinguish between a polyp and a turbinate bone: the former is insensitive and mobile when palpated with a probe (see Figs 11-12 and 11-13). Extensive polyps may protrude from the nose and in extreme cases the nasal bones may be splayed apart producing a frog face (Fig 16-6). The signs and symptoms of nasal polyps are variable because polyps can undergo spontaneous regression without treatment.

Investigations

Positive skin tests are no more common in people with polyps, but a concomitant allergy to house dust or pollen may exist and advice can be given accordingly.

In a child an encephalocele should be excluded (by CT scanning), and a sweat test should be performed to identify cystic fibrosis.

Medical Treatment

Topical Steroids

At least 50% of people with nasal polyps have a good response to topical steroids. Currently, it is not possible to identify the responders before treatment. If the polyps are causing minimal symptoms, it is reasonable to use topical steroids as a first line of management. A 1-month course with review is appropriate.

The most effective method of applying steroid *drops* is in the form of drops administered when the patient is in the head down position (Figs 16-7 and 16-8). In this position, the steroid reaches the target area: the ethmoid cells. After an initial treatment, the patient can change to an aqueous *spray* of topical steroid. The spray needs to be used each day on a prolonged daily basis. (Leaving the spray by the toothbrush is a good reminder.) There are few unwanted effects associated with topical steroid sprays because only a small fraction of the dose is absorbed systemically.

Systemic Steroids

Providing there are no contraindications, systemic steroids have a role in the treatment of severe polyposis and are relatively safe if used in a short reducing dose. The very rare complication of avascular necrosis of the femur can, however, occur even with a short course of systemic steroids.

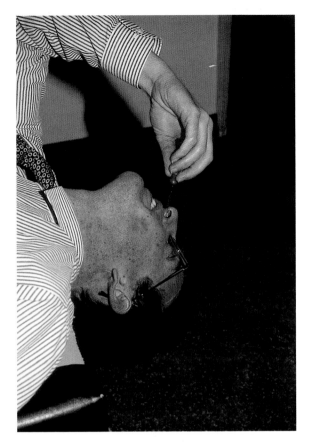

Fig 16-7

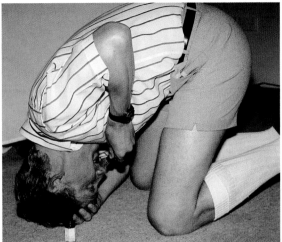

Fig 16-8

Fig 16-8 Another way of administering nasal drops (it is not necessary to wear shorts).

Fig 16-7 One way to administer nasal steroid drops correctly.

Surgical Treatment

Nasal Polypectomy

The majority of patients with polyps require a polypectomy, which clears the bulk of the disease. Topical steroids are then required postoperatively. A nasal polypectomy can be carried out under a local or general anesthetic. With the use of an endoscope, a partial or total ethmoidectomy can be safely performed and in this way the majority of the polyps can be removed. There is some evidence to suggest that endoscopic ethmoidectomy is a more effective treatment than simple nasal polypectomy.

Postoperative Nasal Sprays

Topical steroids given postoperatively reduce the rate of recurrence. The problem is how long to keep the patient on the steroid spray. This will depend on the severity of the polyps, the age of the patient, and how often they have recurred. A minimal time is 3 months.

Key Points:

1. Be suspicious of the unilateral nasal polyp—it may be malignant. Always send it for histology.

2. Most patients presenting with polyps should have them removed using endoscopic techniques. Postoperative topical steroids should be used.

3. Nasal polyps are "like weeds"—they tend to recur; the most effective weed killer is topical steroid.

4. Polyps are rare in children: exclude cystic fibrosis.

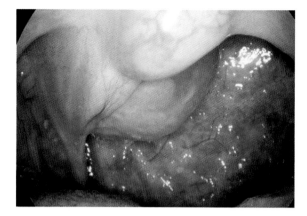

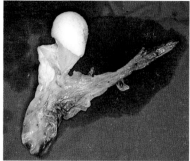

Fig 16-10 Operative specimen of an antrochoanal polyp showing the nasal polyp and its roots from the maxillary sinus.

Fig 16-9 An antrochoanal polyp forms from the maxillary antrum and gradually expands until it hangs down into the postnasal space.

Antrochoanal Polyps

These are unilateral polyps that arise from the lining of a maxillary sinus. The polyp is single and arises in the maxillary antrum. It protrudes through the maxillary ostium and projects backward to the postnasal space (Fig 16-9). The polyp has a dumbell shape because of constriction at the sinus ostium (Fig 16-10). The etiology is unknown and the polyp is benign.

The most common symptom is nasal blockage, which is unilateral unless the polyp is large enough to block both sides of the postnasal space.

Treatment

The treatment is removal via the nose using an endoscope. Antrochoanal polyps can recur.

SEPTAL PERFORATIONS

Etiology

The causes of septal perforations are shown in Table 16-1.

The most common cause of a septal perforation is postsurgical trauma (Fig 16-11). This complication may occur with any type of septal surgery. If the perforation has granulation tissue with it think of Wegener's granuloma or lymphoma. The perforation of syphilis is usually farther back in the bony septum.

Aggressive nose picking and overenthusiastic cautery can both cause perforations. When using silver nitrate, it is wise to cauterize just one side of Little's area at a time.

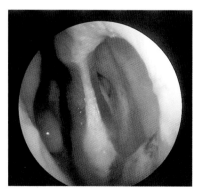

Fig 16-11 Perforation of the septum. Think of the underlying causes!

Table 16-1. Causes of Septal Perforation

1. **Trauma**
   Postsurgery
   Nasal cautery
   Pressure from nasal balloons
   Nose picking

2. **Chronic Infections**
   Syphilis, tuberculosis, leprosy

3. **Malignant Tumors**
   Melanoma, carcinoma, lymphoma

4. **Autoimmune**
   Wegener's, sarcoidosis

5. **Chemical Trauma**
   Cocaine addiction

Clinical Features

A small perforation may present with whistling as the patient breathes in and out, but this is lost as the perforation enlarges. A septal perforation may present with nasal obstruction, because crusting occurs around the edges of the perforation. It may also present with bleeding because crusts become detached leaving vessels exposed. A severe septal perforation leads to collapse and fibrosis, so that the nasal dorsum is depressed (saddle nose).

Treatment

No treatment is required if the perforation is asymptomatic. Saline douches and the application of vaseline to the edges are helpful in combating excessive crusting. Granulation tissue around a perforation should be biopsied.

The surgical closure of a septal perforation is difficult. Many operations are described which rely on transposing mucosal flaps. An alternative is to insert a specially made silastic button into the hole, but this is not tolerated by all patients.

Key Points:

1. Malignant disease and granulomas can present with a perforation, and biopsy of any abnormal tissue should be routine.

2. Aggressive cautery to the nasal septum can result in a septal perforation.

CHAPTER 17

Fractures of the Nose and Midface

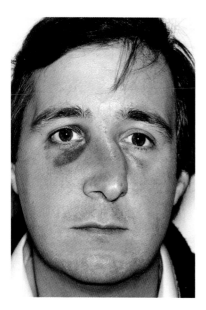

Fig 17-1 A sideways blow from the right has fractured the nose and produced this deformity. Always ensure that the zygoma has not been fractured.

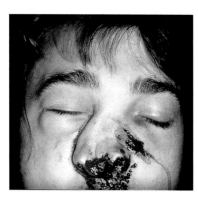

Fig 17-2 A compound nasal fracture.

NASAL FRACTURES

This injury is common in contact sports and fights. If the blow is from the front, the nasal bones may be depressed. Often the blow comes from the side so that the nasal bones are deviated. In children, the possibility of nonaccidental injury may need to be considered

A nasal fracture may be simple (Fig 17-1), or compound (exposed bone or cartilage, Fig 17-2).

Symptoms

The patient complains of nasal deformity, obstruction, and bleeding.

Examination

On examination, the deformity is usually obvious. Careful palpation will reveal whether or not the nasal bones are depressed and which, if any, are deviated. It is important to examine the nasal cavity to see if a septal hematoma is present. Radiography is not required for an isolated nasal fracture.

Treatment

A nasal fracture can be reduced under a local or general anaesthetic. This can be done immediately (ie, before the onset of swelling) or after 7 days when the swelling has subsided.

The deformity is at first accentuated so that the bony fragments are disimpacted. Swinging the nose back toward the midline then reduces the fracture. If a nasal bone is depressed, it can be lifted using an elevator. If the nose is unstable following reduction, a plaster is applied for a week.

Complications of Nasal Fracture

Septal Hematoma

A septal haematoma (Fig 17-3) occurs when there has been a shearing injury stripping the perichondrium from the underlying cartilage. The blood supply to the cartilage comes from the perichondrium and the cartilage may necrose if the hematoma is not drained. If an abscess forms in the hematoma, the destruction of cartilage is accelerated and intracranial sepsis may follow. Cartilage necrosis is disastrous because subsequent fibrosis causes collapse of the nasal bridge ("saddle nose") and gross nasal obstruction.

A septal hematoma can be diagnosed by examination. The septum, which is usually thin and firm, becomes swollen, and palpation with a probe will confirm the swelling is fluctuant. The patient is usually very uncomfortable and often complains of complete nasal obstruction.

A hematoma needs urgent drainage and firm nasal packing so that the perichondrium adheres to the cartilage.

Septal Deviation

It is hard to correct deformed cartilage definitively with simple manipulation as its "springiness" tends to make it dislodge. An elective septoplasty may be required or the operation may be done acutely.

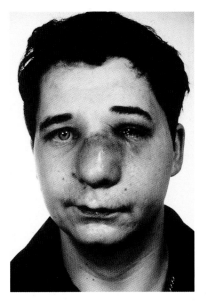

Fig 17-3 This patient developed a septal hematoma followed by a septal abscess.

Nasal Deformity

Nasal fractures are frequently neglected (Fig 17-4). Failure to correct adequately the initial deformity may necessitate difficult secondary procedures later.

Key Points:

1. In a patient with a nasal injury, always examine inside the nose to exclude a septal hematoma. If present, a septal hematoma needs urgent treatment.

2. Nasal fractures may be reduced immediately or after 7-10 days.

3. Adequate initial treatment of fractures will remove the need for difficult reconstructive procedures later.

4. A concomitant fracture of the facial skeleton (eg, of the zygoma) should always be excluded.

5. X-rays of the nasal bones are not necessary in the management of isolated nasal fractures.

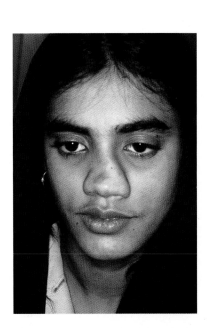

Fig 17-4 This nasal deformity resulted from an untreated nasal fracture. Primary reduction is strongly recommended to prevent the need for difficult secondary reconstruction such as shown here.

TRAUMA TO THE SINUSES AND THE MIDDLE AND LOWER FACE

Fractures of the Zygoma and the Bony Orbit

Combined fractures of these structures are common (Fig 17-5). The mechanism of fracture is usually a blunt violent injury to the lateral part of the face.

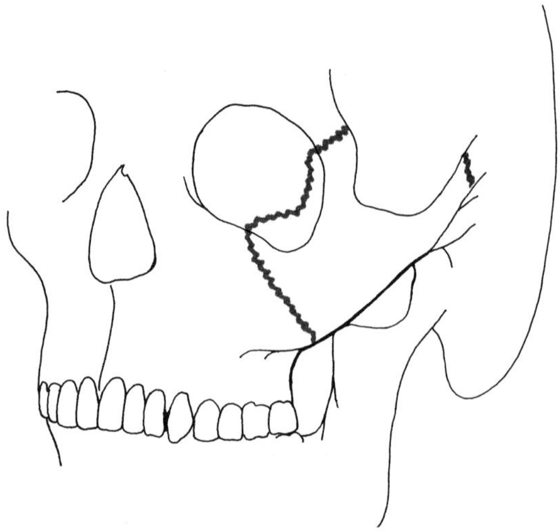

Fig 17-5 The tripod fracture, so named because the fracture line runs through the zygomatic arch, the orbital rim, and the zygomatic process. Check integrity of orbital rim, infra-orbital nerve, and eye movements.

Examination

Inspection may reveal the globe at a slightly lower level than its fellow at the opposite side. Palpate the orbital rim to see if the fracture has produced a step. A depressed maxilla may not be obvious because of soft tissue swelling. There may be parasthesia or numbness in the distribution of the infraorbital nerve. Carefully check the patient's jaw movements. Examination of the eye movements, particularly upward gaze, can detect orbital entrapment.

Treatment

A nondisplaced fracture without any complications does not require treatment. Orbital entrapment, a displaced fracture, or infraorbital nerve damage require reduction.

An uncomplicated fracture of the zygoma simply needs elevation. An unstable fracture may need open reduction and wiring.

Isolated "Blow Out" Fracture of the Orbit

This is often caused by a ball hitting the orbit directly. The squash ball is notorious because it is just the right size to fit in the bony orbit. The floor of the orbit is a weak spot that fractures under pressure and may lead to entrapment of orbital contents. The orbital fat, inferior rectus, and inferior oblique muscles may be trapped.

Such entrapment produces enophthalmus, double vision, and limitation of eye movement.

A radiograph shows a typical "tear drop" sign, which is due to soft tissue trapped in the fracture.

Entrapment requires surgical exploration. The orbital contents are freed and a silastic prosthesis can be placed on the orbital floor to hold the contents in place.

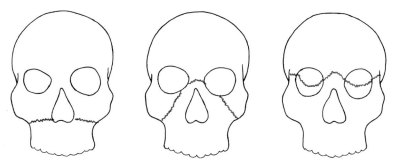

Fig 17-6 Le Fort fractures. Le Fort I: The upper alveolus is detached. Le Fort II: The entire upper jaw is detached; Le Fort III: The facial skeleton is separated from the skull base and may obscure the airway.

Fractures of the Middle Third of the Face

Fractures of the middle third of the face can compromise the airway. These are most commonly transverse and result from direct trauma to the face. Three typical fracture lines were worked out by Le Fort who dropped cement bags from the ramparts of a castle onto cadaver heads (Fig 17-6).

Middle third fractures result from high-speed injuries and this is most likely to occur with motor vehicle accidents. This type of injury is much reduced when seatbelt laws are rigorously applied. Careful history and examination are important. The middle third of the face is inspected and careful palpation around the facial structures is made. It is essential to check jaw movements and mobility of the upper jaw (maxilla). It is important to examine the eye and eye movements.

Management

These patients often have multiple injuries and need urgent resuscitation. The first priority is the airway because the tongue or a mobile maxilla may obstruct it. A useful immediate measure is to pass a Foley catheter into the nasopharynx via the nose. By inflating the balloon and applying traction, the maxilla can be pulled forward. A tracheostomy may be required if endotracheal intubation is unsuccessful.

All patients should have radiographic examinations of the chest, cervical spine, and head. In this way significant chest and spinal fractures will be recognized at the outset.

Air in the cranial cavity indicates a skull base fracture, and a CSF leak is likely to occur. The treatment of spine, chest, or skull fractures will take precedence over the definitive treatment of facial fractures. Reduction and fixation of the facial fractures is undertaken when the patient's condition permits.

Severe fractures may require the combined efforts of neurosurgeons oral-maxillofacial surgeons, and otolaryngologists.

Fractures of the Mandible

With severe fractures of the mandible the priority is to maintain the airway and stop hemorrhage. Considerable force is required to fracture the mandible so it is important not to overlook intracranial or other injury.

Examination

Look and feel both inside and outside the mouth for deformity and malocclusion, and test for labial sensation (inferior dental nerve).

Investigations

An orthopantamogram (OPG) is the most helpful radiograph.

Treatment

Undisplaced fractures with no malocclusion do not require operative treatment. This is usually the case with fractures of the condyle, ascending ramus, and angle of the mandible. Analgesia and antibiotics are sufficient.

A *simple fracture* that reduces easily can be held in place by intermaxillary fixation. A common method of achieving this is to wire the teeth of the maxilla to those of the mandible (eyelet wiring).

An *irreducible fracture* or one that is unstable requires an open reduction and fixation. After reduction the fragments are held in alignment with either wires or an AO plate.

Key Points:

1. In orbital trauma, check the eye movements, palpate the bony orbital rim, and record visual acuity.

2. In patients with facial injury, always check the full range of jaw movements and determine whether or not the upper jaw is mobile. Fractures of the cheek bone (zygoma) are often overlooked.

3. Wear eye protection while playing racquet sports.

CHAPTER 18

Epistaxis

A nose bleed (epistaxis) should never be underestimated—the blood loss can be life-threatening.

In young people the bleeding site is generally on the anterior part of the nasal septum, just behind the columella (Little's area) (Fig 18-1). With increasing age, the site of bleeding moves farther back in the nose. Posterior bleeds are usually more severe and can be difficult to control.

Epistaxis may be due to local or general causes (Table 18-1). Patients with hypertension do not bleed more often, but when an epistaxis occurs, it is more severe. Hypertensives, therefore, account for an increased proportion of hospital admissions for epistaxis.

LOCAL CAUSES OF BLEEDING WITHIN THE NOSE

Nose Picking

The anterior part of the septum (Little's area, also known as Kesselbach's plexus) (see Fig 18-1) is an area where the mucosa

---

Table 18-1. The Causes of Epistaxis

Local Causes
1. **Trauma**
   Nose picking
   Fractures: nasal bones, skull base, sinuses
   Following nasal surgery
2. **Idiopathic**
   Posterior bleeds (>30 yrs)—vessel "degeneration"
3. **Neoplastic**
   Bleeding polyp septum
   Angiofibroma
   Carcinoma—nose, sinuses, postnasal space
   Lymphoma
   Wegener's granuloma
General Causes
1. **Medication**
   Anticoagulants
2. **Hematological disease**
   Familial hereditary telangectasia (Osler's disease)
   Bleeding diatheses

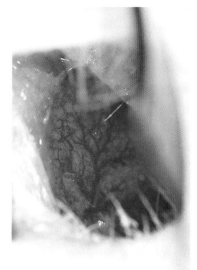

Fig 18-1 Little's area. A rich anastomosis of vessels on the anterior part of the septum. A common site for epistaxis.

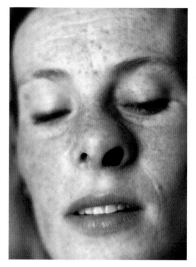

Fig 18-2 Bleeding polyp of the septum (left side). This polyp enlarged during pregnancy.

may dry, particularly if there is a septal deviation. If crusting occurs, the vessels may bleed when the crust is picked away. This type of bleeding is particularly common in childhood. Local anesthetic is applied to the anterior septum and the bleeding point cauterized.

Aging

The posterior bleeds of advancing age are thought to be due to degeneration of blood vessels. The muscular tunica media is replaced with fibrous tissue and calcification occurs in the larger arteries. The bleeding site may be on the posterior septal wall or the lateral wall of the nose.

Bleeding Polyp of the Septum

This is rare. A bleeding polyp of the septum is occasionally seen on the anterior third of the septum (Fig 18-2). This is a red inflammatory mass, which is thought to be caused by mechanical irritation and is treated by excision.

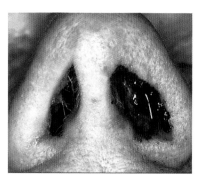

Fig 18-3 Epistaxis. The patient presented with left-sided nose bleeds. Examination confirmed a malignant melanona.

Neoplasms

A malignant lesion in the nose or sinuses often presents with a serosanguinous discharge rather than fresh blood (Fig 18-3). One of the presenting symptoms of a nasopharyngeal carcinoma is epistaxis. An angiofibroma is an uncommon tumor that occurs in adolescent males and arises in the posterior part of the nose. It presents with profuse and recurrent epistaxes.

N.B. *Beware unilateral bloody discharge.*

Trauma

Facial trauma can give rise to persistent epistaxis, particularly where fragments of the fracture overlap. When the fracture is reduced the epistaxis tends to settle.

SYSTEMIC CAUSES OF EPISTAXIS

Familial Hereditary Telangiectasia (Osler's Disease)

This is a systemic disease (Fig 18-4) in which there is a deficiency in the endothelial layer of blood vessels. Telangiectases are present on the face, lips, buccal mucosa, and tongue. Bleeding can occur at several points throughout the aero-digestive tract. The epistaxes can be difficult to control. Skin grafting of the septum, laser treatment, or estrogen therapy may be needed.

Oral Anticoagulants and Blood Dyscrasias

Control of the epistaxis in these patients requires collaboration with the patient's hematologist.

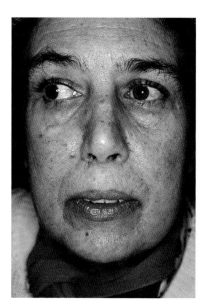

Fig 18-4 Hereditary hemorrhagic telangiectasia (Osler's disease). The patient experienced profuse nose bleeding. Note the facial telangiectasia. The mainstay of treatment is estrogen therapy.

THE MANAGEMENT OF EPISTAXIS

History

The patient may need immediate resuscitation but, generally it is possible to take a history to elicit local or systemic causes for the epistaxis and to assess the amount of blood loss. Always enquire about the patient's medications (anticoagulants, aspirin ingestion, etc).

General Measures

It is important to have a positive attitude and to appear calm and in control. It may be a life-threatening condition which the patient and possibly the nurse have never encountered, but (hopefully) *you have.*

Practical measures are the same as for any patient following blood loss. Depending on the severity of the bleed, vital signs must be monitored. Blood should be taken for complete blood count, cross matching, and coagulation studies, as indicated. Intravenous fluid replacement may be needed.

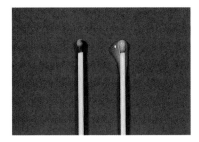

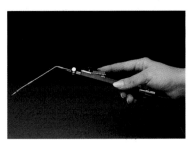

Fig 18-5 Silver nitrate cautery. On the wet mucous membrane, the silver nitrate is converted to nitric acid (on the right).

Fig 18-6 Electrocautery. To prevent burns to the skin, it should only be turned on inside the nose when it is in contact with the bleeding point. Before removing the cautery, switch off the current.

Examination

The doctor should wear gloves, goggles, and an apron to protect from contact with blood. Any blood clots in the nose need to be removed (ask the patient to blow the nose, or use a sucker). The nose should be anesthetized with lignocaine and adrenaline solution or cocaine spray.

Electric or Chemical Cautery

Bleeding vessels can be cauterized with silver nitrate or electrocautery after local anesthesia. If silver nitrate (Fig 18-5) is used it is imperative to cauterize around the vessel and leave the stick in contact with the mucosa for at least 10 seconds. Care is needed to prevent any nitric acid running out onto the skin, which can cause a chemical burn.

Electrocautery (Fig 18-6) has its dangers. It is easy to burn the skin of the nose if one is not extremely careful. Always test the cautery *before* inserting it in the patient's nose. *Do not introduce a red hot cautery into the nose—this terrifies the patient and makes a burn more likely.* Switch on the cautery only when the tip is actually on the bleeding site and switch it off before removing it from the nostril.

If there is no obvious bleeding site in the front of the nose, the posterior nose can be examined with the nasopharyngoscope or the microscope.

Packs and Balloons

If a bleeding point cannot be identified and controlled, a nasal pack may be necessary.

Merocel nasal tampons (Figs 18-7 and 18-8) are easy to insert into the nose and swell on contact with blood. Merocel packs

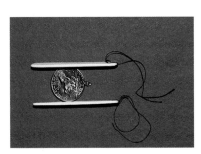

Fig 18-7 Merocel packs are thin and stiff and are therefore easy to insert without the aid of a headlight or suction.

should be in the bag of every family practitioner because they can be inserted without the help of a headlight and forceps.

If Merocel packing fails, bismuth iodoform paraffin paste (BIPP) is commonly used to pack the nose (Fig 18-9). A ribbon gauze impregnated with adrenaline and cocaine is also suitable.

A balloon is an alternative to a pack and various types are available (Fig 18-10). Once the nose is packed or a balloon inserted, hospital admission is usually advised in case the pack dislodges and obstructs the airway. A nasal pack may cause a reflex hypoxemia, which can be important in patients with respiratory insufficiency. Depending on the severity of the bleed it is usual to leave a pack or balloon in place for 24 to 48 hours. Antibiotic cover is advisable.

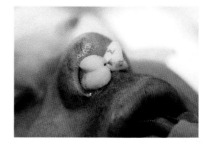

Fig 18-8 Contact with liquid causes the Merocel packs to expand.

Bedrest and sedation are an important part of treatment for severe epistaxis. An elevated blood pressure usually settles with bedrest. If the diastolic pressure remains high the advice of a physician is essential. A summary of the management of epistaxis is given in Table 18-2.

Recalcitrant Epistaxis

A persistent or recurrent epistaxis presents a challenge. The exact method of dealing with the problem will depend on the individual patient but a number of options are available.

Firm Packing of the Posterior Nose

This is combined with packing the anterior nose and requires a general anesthetic.

Vasopressin

Synthetic forms of vasopressin (antidiuretic hormone) can be applied topically on a nasal pack or can be given systemically by intravenous injection. Its use is restricted to severe epistaxis.

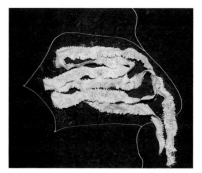

Fig 18-9 Nasal packing. Remove the blood clot and anesthetize the nose with cocaine or lignocaine. Insert the pack by building it up in layers from the floor of the nose upward. Roughly 1 meter of packing can be inserted into the average nostril. Good light and suction are still required.

Table 18-2. The Treatment of Epistaxis

General Measures	Monitor vital signs
	Blood for FBC, cross match, coagulation studies
	Intravenous infusion
Local Measures	Topical anesthetic spray
	Cautery (electric or chemical)
	Packing: BIPP, balloons, tampons
	Vessel ligation (external carotid, maxillary or ethmoidal arteries)
	Septal surgery

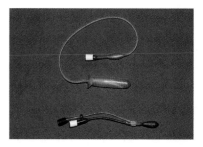

Fig 18-10 Examples of nasal balloons that can be used to control epistaxis.

Ligation of Feeding Vessels

The majority of the blood supply to the nose comes from the sphenopalatine artery, which is a branch of the maxillary artery. The sphenopalatine artery enters the nasal cavity through a foramen that lies behind the maxillary ostium. With an endoscope it is relatively easy to reach this artery and ligate it. This is becoming the method of choice for severe or recurrent epistaxis. Alternatively, the maxillary artery can be clipped as it courses behind the maxillary antrum. Finally, the external carotid artery can be ligated in the neck.

Bleeding predominantly from the superior part of the nose requires ligation of the ethmoidal vessels on the medial wall of the orbit. This is a simple procedure performed via an external ethmoidectomy approach.

Septoplasty

This helps to gain access to the bleeding site. The operation itself can sometimes prevent recurrent epistaxis because the vessels become fibrosed after mucosal flaps have been raised and replaced.

Embolization of Feeding Blood Vessels

If the patient is actively bleeding, a skilled radiologist may be able to demonstrate the bleeding vessel by cannulating the aterial system and injecting contrast. The offending vessel can then be embolized with polyvinyl particles. Embolization is usually reserved for severe epistaxis that has not been controlled by other means, but it may be difficult in the elderly if there is atherosclerosis.

Key Points:

1. Epistaxis can cause life-threatening blood loss. Systemic and local measures are necessary in the management of these patients.

2. There may be a local or systemic cause for the epistaxis.

3. It is safer to admit patients to hospital following insertion of a nasal pack. A pack can dislodge and become aspirated.

4. Severe epistaxis may require vessel ligation or embolization.

CHAPTER 19

Facial Pain and Headache

The management of facial pain is a challenge, both diagnostically and therapeutically. The occurrence of referred pain and the complex nerve supply to the head and neck mean that a thorough history and examination are paramount for the accurate diagnosis of facial pain. If a clear diagnosis cannot be established, then beware of misguided attempts at treatment, especially surgery. Somatic and psychogenic pain overlap and few patients suffer exclusively from one or the other.

The nerve fibers responsible for facial pain mainly travel in the spinal tract in the brain stem and are unmyelinated. The spinal tract receives contributions from the trigeminal nerve (V) and the VIIth, IXth, and Xth cranial nerves. Afferent fibers from the cervical spine also merge into the tract. There is a large amount of crossover between afferent fibers. The result is that facial pain generally is poorly localized and incorrect central interpretation (referred pain) is common.

There are many examples of *referred pain* in the head and neck, eg, irritation of the cranial nerve IX (post-tonsillectomy) causes referred otalgia. A laryngeal carcinoma can also present with referred otalgia. Both cranial nerves IX and X have branches that supply the ear as well as the pharynx and larynx, respectively (Fig 19-1).

History

The history is very important and a good idea of the cause of the pain or headache can often be obtained once the frequency, duration, severity, and associated symptoms have been established together with the overall time course.

A useful formula:

$$\text{Headache or pain} = \frac{\text{F.D.S} + \text{A}}{\text{T}}$$

Where
F = freqency
D = duration
S = severity
A = associated symptoms
T = overall time course

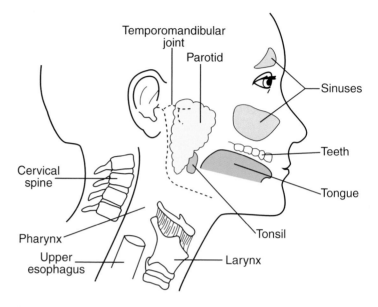

Fig 19-1 All of the above sites can give rise to referred otalgia.

Migraine, for example, often has prodromal symptoms, a gradual onset, and slow buildup and it typically lasts between 4 and 72 hours; whereas pain or headache that remains constant for many months and is not associated with other symptoms seldom has a physical basis.

Ask about:

1. The site of the pain and its radiation.

2. The periodicity of the pain.

3. The pattern of the pain and how it progresses.

4. The duration of the pain.

5. Precipitating factors.

6. Factors that relieve the pain.

7. What treatment has already been tried.

EXAMINATION

A full otoneurological examination needs to be undertaken. Often no abnormal signs are found, but if there are, further investigation is required.

Patients with facial pain or headache present to family practitioners and various specialists including otolaryngologists. A classification based on an otolaryngology perspective is given in Table 19-1.

Table 19-1. A Classification of Facial Pain

Condition	Comment
Local Causes of Facial Pain	
Rhinological	Aim for definite diagnosis
Otalgia	Beware referred cause
Ophthalmic	Don't miss glaucoma
Temporomandibular joint	Possible malocclusion
Dental pain	OPG radiograph
Cervical spine	MRI
Tension Headache	Common, no signs, anxious/depressed patient
Vascular Causes	
Temporal arteritis	Diagnose and treat to avoid loss of vision
Migraine	Prodromal symptoms, slow buildup, 4-72 hours
Cluster headaches	Episodes occur in bouts
Primary Neuralgias	
Trigeminal, glossopharyngeal	No objective signs
Secondary Neuralgias	
(eg, Multiple sclerosis or tumor)	Objective signs
Causalgia (Reflex sympathetic dystrophy)	Difficult to treat
Atypical Facial Pain	A definite entity

PAIN AND HEADACHE FROM A RHINOLOGICAL CAUSE

Patients often think or have been told that they have "sinus" pain and sometimes they are right!

Acute infective rhinosinusitis is painful. Typically the pain is worse on bending. It is usually localized over the infected sinus, although infection in the sphenoid can give rise to pain over the temples or vertex. Infection in the maxillary antrum may cause pain in the upper teeth. Infection is not the only cause of rhinosinusitis and mucosal swelling from whatever cause can lead to sinus obstruction, which presents with blockage, congestion, and sometimes pain. A blocked sinus alone (without any infection) can certainly produce severe pain as occurs in the sinus headaches associated with barotrauma.

Typically chronic rhinosinusitis presents with obstruction, postnasal drip, and congestion around the eyes. The patient may describe a feeling of blockage high up under the nasal bones even though the nasal airway seems adequate. An individual with chronic sinusitis may have acute exacerbations of pain that particularly occur with upper respiratory tract infections.

Although a patient with rhinosinusitis may complain of facial swelling, it is rare to see this and, if present, it suggests a dental infection or carcinoma (see Fig 20-7).

OTALGIA

Otalgia may be due to pathology within the ear or be due to referred pain. Otitis externa, otitis media, and mastoiditis have specific signs and symptoms. The most common causes of referred otalgia are impacted molars, tonsillitis (including tonsillectomy), dental infection, and temperomandibular dysfunction. Tumors of the oral cavity, pharynx, or larynx may also result in earache and should always be considered.

OPHTHALMIC PAIN

Refractive errors and various ocular palsies may be associated with pain in the eyes and generalized headache. Glaucoma can present severe orbital pain and headache, and the patient may see halos around lights.

Vision can deteriorate rapidly so an early diagnosis and treatment are required.

Orbital pain can be caused by uveitis, keratitis, and dry-eye syndrome. The red, swollen proptosed eye is due either to a preseptal infection or to an infection that may lie behind the septum, in which case it is ethmoiditis (p174).

TEMPOROMANDIBULAR JOINT DYSFUNCTION

This usually occurs in young adults. In 90% of cases the pain is unilateral and often there is a malocclusion which puts strain on the joint capsule.

A plain radiograph of the joint is usually normal. The pain is described as a deep, dull ache around the joint and the ear. The pain may radiate down the neck or up into the temple. Otalgia tinnitus may also occur. It may be related to chewing but is not always so. The pain is thought to arise because of spasm in the pterygoid muscles. Look for malocclusion or crossbite and palpate intraorally for joint tenderness.

Treatment involves reassurance, special exercises, and correction of malocclusion with dental splints.

PAIN OF DENTAL ORIGIN

Defects in the enamel of a tooth may produce sharp, well-localized pain. When the pulp of the tooth is infected, the pain is dull and poorly localized. Once the peridontium is involved, the pain again becomes well localized and at this stage there will usually be swelling and erythema of the gingivae.

Pain of dental origin can sometimes be difficult to diagnose, as occasionally the only finding is localized tenderness on chewing. The pain usually presents locally but it may also be referred to the ear.

Radiological examination, particularly the orphopantamogram, is useful to detect a root abscess. Caries, periapical disease, peridontal abscesses, osteomyeilitis, fractures, and neoplasms in the maxilla and mandible are all causes of facial pain.

PAIN FROM CERVICAL SPINE DISORDERS

These are very common and range from a mild spondylosis to severe arthritic change narrowing the foramen in the cervical spine. Even with moderate changes in the cervical spine, occipital pain, backache, or pain radiating down the arm may be present. An MRI scan is diagnostic. Physiotherapy is most helpful.

TENSION HEADACHE

This is a common condition. The patient describes a tightness or pressure around the head (temples, vertex, and suboccipital regions). The intensity is variable and the patient is often anxious and /or depressed. The headache may last for several days and may only partly respond to analgesics. There will be no accompanying neurological signs. Reassurance and low dose tricylics (amitryptilline) may be helpful.

FACIAL PAIN AND HEADACHE FROM A VASCULAR CAUSE

Temporal Arteritis

Temporal arteritis usually occurs in patients over 50 and is more common in women. This disease is not restricted to the temporal artery, but is a generalized inflammation throughout the arteries in the head and neck. Typically the patient describes a deep, boring pain in the temporal region. The temporal artery itself is tender on palpation and thickened. There are systemic signs with a raised temperature. If left untreated 40% of patients will develop visual loss due to involvement of the ophthalmic artery. It is also possible for the patient to present with unilateral blindness.

The erythrocyte sedimentation rate (ESR) is almost always raised. A biopsy of the temporal artery reveals the giant cell arteritis that obliterates the lumen.

Treatment is with steroids and this should not be delayed.

Migraine

Migraine presents in a variety of ways and affects 10% of adults. It classically presents with prodromal symptoms, which include visual disturbance, nausea, and paresthesias. There is often a family history. Migraine can be induced by tiredness, stress, climate change, and certain dietary substances (eg, chocolate, cheese). It is thought to be caused by transient vasoconstriction of cerebral arteries followed by vasodilation. The process sweeps across an area of cortex, hence visual disturbance may be followed by parasthesia, then vomiting and headache. Migraine affecting the vertebrobasilar system may be accompanied by vertigo and ataxia.

Characteristically there is a slow buildup and the whole episode lasts between 4 and 72 hours.

Treatment is by avoiding the triggering factors and with medication aimed at either the acute episode or prophylactic cover.

For acute symptoms: Simple analgesics (paracetamol) and anti-emetics should be tried first followed by either ergotamine derivates or sumatriptan, a 5 HT1 antagonist.

For prophylaxis: Pizotifen, an antihistamine and serotonin antagonist; beta blockers; or tricyclics medication are all effective.

CLUSTER HEADACHES (PERIODIC MIGRAINOUS NEURALGIA)

The clinical syndrome consists of severe unilateral pain with a blocked nose. Typically the episodes occur in bouts, hence the name "cluster" headache. The pain is intense and lasts for 2 to 3 hours. The patient may be woken by the pain. There is then a long period of remission before a similar bout of recurrent headache. Cluster headaches differ from classical migraine in that they are much more common in males. The pain also tends to be constant, usually in the region of one eye.

Alcohol should be avoided and ergotamine derivates or sumatriptan can be used during the cluster period.

NEURALGIAS

A neuralgia is a pain in the area of distribution of a sensory nerve.

Primary Neuralgias

These occur in certain cranial nerves (trigeminal and glossopharyngeal) and are not accompanied by objective signs of impaired nerve function.

A primary neuralgia is characterized by a sharp severe pain, rather like a stab with a knife, that lasts for a few seconds. There may be trigger zones that provoke the pain, but there are no objective signs of impaired nerve function.

Many explanations have been proposed to explain primary neuralgia. It is thought to be similar to epilepsy in that a sudden irregular discharge of nerve impulses occurs.

The quality of the pain and its distribution are the hallmarks of the diagnosis. The pain is usually unilateral. Paroxysms of pain occur in cycles and last for weeks or even months. The pain is so severe that grimaces of the face occur (medieval gargoyles may have been modeled on patients who had trigeminal neuralgia!).

Trigeminal Neuralgia (Tic Doloureux)

Trigeminal neuralgia has an incidence of 5 per 100,000 per year. It is more common in women and the peak age for presentation is between 50 and 60 years. The pain is restricted to the area supplied by the 3 branches of the nerve. The maxillary and mandibular branches are most commonly affected. There is often a trigger area. For example, the patient describes touching or brushing the teeth as the trigger which sets off the pain. Many patients have had unnecessary dental extractions and sinus washouts before the diagnosis is made.

Glossopharyngeal Neuralgia

This is much rarer than trigeminal neuralgia. It follows the distribution of the glossopharyngeal nerve which carries sensation from the pharynx and tonsils, posterior third of the tongue, eustachian tube, middle ear, and external auditory meatus. It is in this distribution that pain is felt and paroxysms are triggered by swallowing, chewing, or yawning. The trigger zones tend to be the tonsils and pharyngeal wall.

Thorough investigation is required to exclude a secondary neuralgia before a diagnosis of primary neuralgia is made. This may involve radiology of the skull base to exclude nerve compression.

Treatment

Antiepileptic drugs (eg, carbamazepine) are usually effective at controlling primary neuralgias. The carbamazepine is started in a low dosage and gradually increased. Gaba pentene is useful in patients who do not respond to carbamazepine. Surgical treatments range from local nerve avulsion to ablation of the sensory ganglion. The help of a pain clinic can be invaluable.

Secondary Neuralgias

This may present like a primary neuralgia initially, but then objective signs of nerve pathology occur. A pathological process can be demonstrated. A common finding would be paresthesia and numbness in the distribution of the nerve involved. The most common causes over the age of 40 years would be a tumor, or aneurysm, whereas under the age of 40 years multiple sclerosis is the most common cause.

Pain in the distribution of a cranial or spinal nerve accompanied by signs of nerve impairment needs complete investigation to find the underlying pathology. A thorough examination can be supplemented by CT or MRI scans.

CAUSALGIA (REFLEX SYMPATHETIC DYSTROPHY)

This occurs when there has been injury to a nerve. The pain is typically a burning pain and it may be accompanied by autonomic changes in the skin. It is thought to be due to disturbed autonomic afferents and sympathetic blockade may relieve the condition.

ATYPICAL FACIAL PAIN

This is a diagnosis in its own right. It should only be made when organic causes have been excluded. Psychological factors play a major role in this condition. The pain is usually severe and persistent and it may be associated with other features of depression. The pain cannot be explained on an anatomical basis and often occurs every day. Rarely are there precipitating factors and it is not relieved by analgesia. It is more common in women over the age of 40. No physical signs of cranial nerve involvement can be detected. It can be a difficult problem to treat, although tricyclic antidepressants may help.

Key Points:

1. Pain in the head, neck, or face can be very difficult to diagnose.

2. CT or MRI scans are not a substitute for thorough history-taking and physical examination.

3. If in doubt, consider referral to a pain clinic rather than surgery.

CHAPTER 20

Tumors of the Nose and Sinuses

There is a wide histological variety of nasal and sinus tumors (Table 20-1). Most are benign, with malignant nasal and sinus tumors accounting for less than 3% of head and neck malignancy. Most nasal tumors present in a similar way and biopsy is required to exclude malignancy. *Always remember that a unilateral polyp or nasal mass in an adult needs removal for histological examination.*

BENIGN TUMORS

Inverting Papilloma (Ringertz Tumor): Rare But Important

The usual presentation is with a unilateral nasal polyp (Figs 20-1 and 20-2). The papilloma arises from within the nose, the ethmoids, or the maxillary sinus. The patient has nasal obstruction and epistaxis is common. The tumor is benign but causes *extensive local destruction.* There is a very small risk of malignant change. Radiological assessment with a CT scan is required. The treatment is removal of all of the tumor either endoscopically or via a lateral rhinotomy approach.

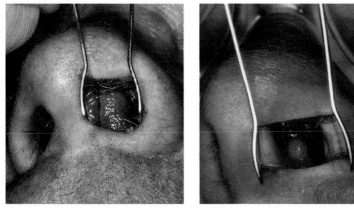

Fig 20-1 This is a unilateral polyp that looks fibrous. It was an inverting papilloma (Ringertz tumor), a benign but locally destructive tumor.

Fig 20-2 A benign nasal polyp for comparison. These polyps were bilateral.

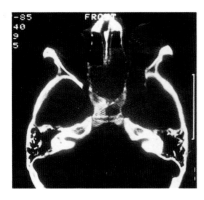

Fig 20-3 A CT scan showing a tumor in the posterior nose of a young adolescent male. This highly vascular tumor was a "juvenile angiofibroma."

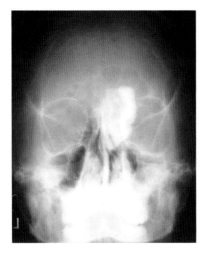

Fig 20-4 An osteoma—common benign tumor of the sinuses.

Key Points:

1. Frequent heavy nose bleeds in an adolescent male should suggest a diagnosis of angiofibroma.

2. A unilateral nasal polyp in an adult should be biopsied.

Juvenile Angiofibroma: Rare But Important (Fig 20-3)

Pathology

This tumor occurs almost exclusively in adolescent males (ages 10-25 years) and arises from the posterior nose (pterygoid plates). The proportions of angiomatous tissue and fibrous tissue vary. The tumor is benign but undergoes expansive growth.

Symptoms

Nasal obstruction, purulent nasal discharge, and frequent epistaxes. Obstruction of the eustachian tube may cause a conductive deafness. Extension to the skull base leads to cranial nerve involvement.

Diagnosis

The diagnosis can often be made from the history. Frequent and heavy epistaxes in a young male are highly suspicious. The tumor will be visible on nasendoscopy.

Imaging

Plain lateral radiographs demonstrate a mass extending from the posterior nose into the postnasal space. CT and MRI scans should give exceptionally good definition of the tumor. Angiography will demonstrate the blood vessels feeding the tumor and allow them to be embolized.

Treatment

The treatment of these tumors is controversial. The most usual treatment is surgical removal. Preoperative embolization reduces the operative bleeding. In some centers radiotherapy is used.

Osteomas

Osteomas are common benign tumors and may be an incidental finding on a sinus radiograph (Fig 20-4). They are most common in the frontal sinus. The osteoma is usually asymptomatic but may cause headache and local tenderness over the sinus. Chronic sinusitis or a mucocele may develop if the ostium becomes obstructed. A frontal osteoma can displace the eye downwards and outwards. A well-demarcated calcified opacity with smooth edges (benign features) is seen on the plain radiograph. If an osteoma causes problems the treatment is complete removal. Large tumors may need craniofacial surgery.

MALIGNANT TUMORS OF THE NOSE AND SINUSES

External Nose

Primary tumors of the external nose include basal cell carcinoma (BCC), squamous cell carcinoma (SCC), and malignant melanoma. These tumors are related to sun exposure.

Basal Cell Carcinoma (BCC)

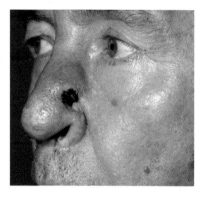

Fig 20-5 A basal cell carcinoma. The rolled edges are typical.

Basal cell carcinoma starts as a firm nodule that increases in size. The growth rate is slow. The tumor then ulcerates (Fig 20-5) and infiltrates into the underlying tissue. The degree of ulceration can be relatively small, but the extension into surrounding tissues can be considerable. Basal cell carcinomas usually do not metastasize. Their hallmark is gross local destruction. Troublesome areas are the columella and eyelids.

Treatment is by wide excision followed by immediate or delayed reconstruction. The prognosis of these tumors is good provided the tumor is excised with clear margins.

Squamous Cell Carcinoma (SCC)

Squamous cell carcinoma is a common tumor of the external nose. Its growth rate is rapid and it ulcerates to form a crater (Fig 20-6). Regional lymph node metastases occur early. The treatment is total excision and this may be combined with radiotherapy. A radical neck dissection is required if there is neck node involvement.

Certain clinical features help distinguish between a BCC and an SCC. The former has a rolled edge and a slow growth rate, but a definitive diagnosis can only be made by histology.

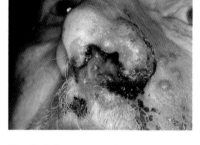

Fig 20-6 Squamous cell carcinoma. Note the raised, everted edges (unlike Fig 20-5).

Malignant Melanoma

This tumour is 40 times more common in Caucasian populations living in the tropics than in those living in temperate zones. It can occur at any age. Ten percent of malignant melanomas occur in the head and neck. The tumor may arise from a pre-existent pigmented mole, but this is not always the case. Suspicious symptoms include an increase in the size of a mole, change in the color, and bleeding. Spread to the lymph nodes is common. The prognosis is determined by the depth and extent of tumor and the patient's immune response.

The mainstay of treatment is rapid and complete excision of the tumor. Nodal involvement may necessitate a radical neck dissection.

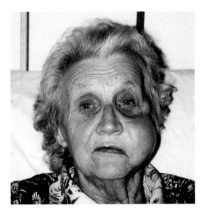

Fig 20-7 Patients with sinusitis frequently complain of swelling but, if the examiner can actually see swelling, there is likely to be underlying dental infection or tumor. This patient had carcinoma of the maxillary antrum.

Malignant Tumors of the Nasal Cavities and Sinuses

Nasal and sinus malignancies make up only 3% of head and neck tumors. A general practitioner may only see one in a lifetime. Sinuses are capacious and can harbor a large tumor silently (Fig 20-7). Nasal and sinus malignancies have a poor prognosis with a 30% to 50% 5-year survival rate.

Histology

A wide variety of histological types of tumor are encountered in the sinuses. The most common is squamous cell carcinoma (SCC), followed by adenocarcinoma, adenoid cystic carcinoma, and malignant melanoma.

Etiology

Only the adenocarcinoma has a known etiology. An increased occurrence of the tumor was noted in furniture makers who worked with hardwoods. The hardwood dust is inhaled, and as 90% of the inspiratory airflow passes the ostiomeatal complex, this is where the carcinoma develops.

Clinical Features

A tumor arising in the nasal cavity is most likely to present with epistaxis and nasal blockage, whereas an ethmoidal tumor is more likely to present with orbital and or neurological symptoms as well as nasal symptoms (Figs 20-8 and 20-9). Only 10% of tumors have palpable neck nodes on first presentation. The lymph drains predominantly to the retropharyngeal and deep cervical nodes, making palpation difficult.

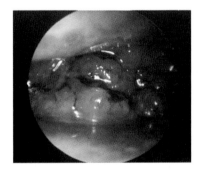

Fig 20-8 This unilateral polyp was a nonpigmented melanoma arising from the ethmoid sinuses. The patient had nasal and orbital problems.

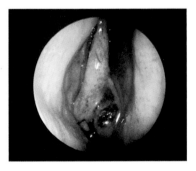

Fig 20-9 This bleeding, unilateral nasal polyp is a carcinoma rising in the maxillary antrum. The patient's main symptoms and signs were nasal.

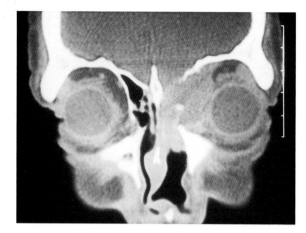

Fig 20-10

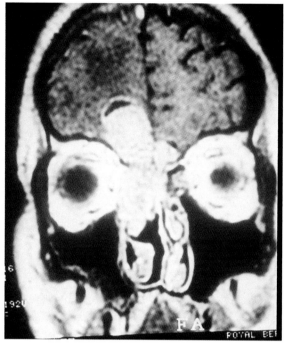

Fig 20-10 A CT scan of a sinus carcinoma demonstrating bony destruction.

Fig 20-11 An MRI of a sinus malignancy delineates the soft tissue.

Fig 20-11

Management

A careful history and examination followed by radiological examination with CT and MRI is required. CT readily demonstrates bony destruction and the MRI delineates the soft tissues (Figs 20-10 and 20-11). Endoscopic techniques usually allow a biopsy to be taken. Histological techniques including immunocytochemistry are able to distinguish the various types of carcinoma from lymphoma.

Treatment

No single treatment is effective. Surgery combined with radiotherapy has produced the best results. Although a good initial response to chemotherapy is often encouraging, it has rarely been shown to increase survival.

The standard surgical approaches for sinus and nasal malignancies are the craniofacial approach and midfacial degloving (p122). The surgical goal is an *en bloc* resection of the entire tumor. At times this may mean removing the contents of the orbit. Osteointegration techniques can help restore cosmesis after such operations (Figs 20-12 and 20-13). Reconstruction of dural or palatal defects may require free flap transfer and often a dental prosthesis is required.

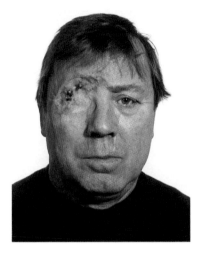

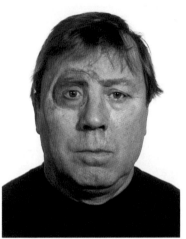

Fig 20-12 Patient with an exenterated orbit. In this case the patient lost his eye because of trauma.

Fig 20-13 Small titanium studs are placed in the rim of the orbit so that a prosthetic eye can be attached. This technique is known as osteo-integration and has many applications.

Lymphoma

Generalized Lymphomas

Generalized lymphonas of both the Hodgkin's and non-Hodgkin's type do occasionally appear in the nose. The local symptoms consist of nasal obstruction, epistaxis, and a mass within the nose. Often there is lymph node involvement at other sites.

Peripheral T Cell (Malignant Lymphona)

This lymphoma behaves differently. These tumors are rare, grow slowly, and, if left untreated, will cause gross destruction of the middle of the face. Immunocytochemistry techniques have identified this lesion as a T cell malignant lymphoma (previously it has been confused with Wegener's). A T cell lymphoma is totally different from Wegener's; there is no systemic involvement. but there is gross local destruction of all the facial tissues. When biospsy material from a T cell lymphoma is examined, there are colonies of T cells but no granulomas and giant cells (cf. Wegener's)

The treatment for a T cell lymphoma is radical radiotherapy, which is usually successful.

Key Points:

1. A unilateral nasal polyp or mass in an adult should always be biopsied.

2. Facial swelling is more often associated with tumor than sinusitis.

3. Woodworkers are at risk of developing ethmoidal adenocarcinoma.

4. The most common tumor of the sinuses is squamous cell carcinoma.

5. Lesions previously called "lethal midline granuloma" or "Stewart's granuloma" were misnamed. These are definitely malignant lymphomas and are totally unrelated to Wegener's granuloma.

Table 20-1. Classification of Nasal and Sinus Tumors

Benign	Malignant
Papilloma	Squamous cell carcinoma
Juvenile angiofibroma	Adenocarcinoma
Inverting papilloma (Ringertz)	Melanoma
Osteomas	Adenoidcystic carcinoma
	Lymphoma
	Rhabdomyosarcoma (childhood)

CHAPTER 21

Specific Infections and Nonspecific Granulomas of the Nose

SPECIFIC INFECTIONS

Each type of specific infection has characteristic features. The diagnosis can be difficult but can usually be determined from the history and pathological examination. Specific antimicrobial treatment is then given.

Fungal Infections

Aspergillus is the fungus that principally infects the nose and sinuses. There is a high incidence of fungal infection in immunocompromised individuals. It is important to think about the possibility of fungal infection in diabetic patients and in patients whose symptoms do not respond quickly to medical treatment. A fungal mass has characteristic areas of calcification on CT scans (Fig 21-1). The treatment is usually local clearance with systemic antifungal medication being reserved for severe cases.

AIDS

A granular rhinitis may be seen. Karposi's sarcoma can occur in the nose. There is usually evidence of HIV elsewhere in the body.

Tuberculosis

The infection may be primary but is usually secondary to mycobacteria in the lungs. There may be nodules or ulcer and the cartilaginous parts of the nose are affected. *Lupus vulgaris* is an indolent and chronic form of tuberculous infection that affects the skin and mucous membranes.

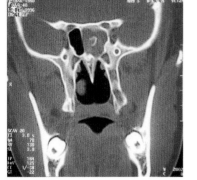

Fig 21-1 A fungal mass within the sphenoid sinus has characteristic areas of calcification on CT scan. This patient presented with a severe "centralized" headache.

Syphilis

Nasal syphilis is now uncommon. It is caused by infection with *Treponema pallidum.* It can occur at any age. The primary chancre can appear on or in the nose and secondary syphilis can present with rhinitis, but it is the tertiary stage that is most frequently encountered in the nose.

The lesion is the gumma which invades mucous membranes and bone. Frequently there is a perforation in the posterior bony septum and the nose may be saddled.

Leprosy

Leprosy is still an important disease in the tropics. The nose is frequently involved in leprosy. Nodules form on the mucous membrane and then the cartilaginous septum is destroyed. Leprosy is caused by the bacillus *Mycobacterium leprae* and the most effective treatment is still diamenodythenal sulphone (dapsone).

NONSPECIFIC GRANULOMAS

Wegener's Granulomatosis (Figs 21-2, 21-3, and 21-4)

This is a systemic disease that is characterized by necrotizing granulomas in the respiratory tract and kidneys together with a

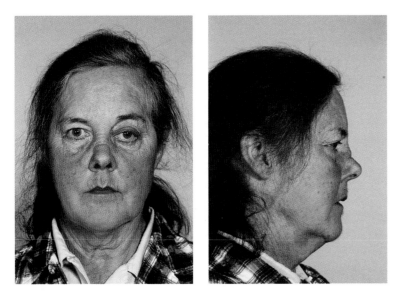

Fig 21-2a   **Fig 21-2b**

Fig 21-2 a. Patient with Wegener's granulomatosis. This is characterized by necrotizing granulomas in the respiratory tract and renal system. **b.** Cartilage and bone is destroyed, which leads to nasal saddling.

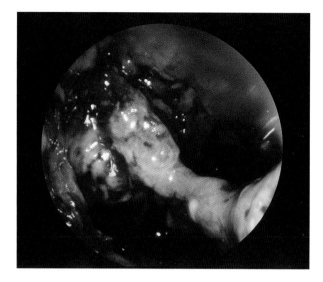

Fig 21-3 Photograph inside the patient's nose (from Fig 21-1a). Most of the "nasal furniture" has disappeared.

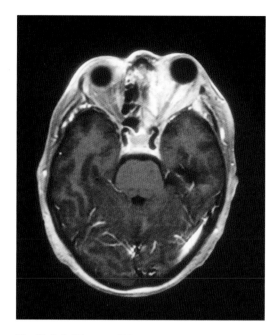

Fig 21-4 A CT scan of Wegener's granuloma involving the orbit.

generalized vasculitis. The etiology is not known, although it is suspected to be an abnormal immune response to an infective agent. The disease is limited to the head and neck region in 45% of patients. The patient often initially presents to the otolaryngologist. *It is easy to miss the diagnosis!* The patient feels unwell, and may have chronic sinus symptoms that persist despite medical treatment. Typical symptoms are nasal stuffiness, watery discharge, and crusting. With time the cartilage and bone "dissolve" and the nose saddles (see Fig 21-2). Orbital involvement is common and presents with proptosis and inflammation. The disease can affect any site in the respiratory tract. Vasculitis within the renal system is common and 10% of patients have CNS and/or skin involvement.

On examination look for crusting, granulations, and destruction (eg, septal perforation). There is often a terrible smell to the nasal discharge. The differential diagnosis is with all forms of granulomas within the nose (eg, sarcoidosis, turberculosis, leprosy, and fungal infections). T cell lymphomas occur within the nose and initially may resemble Wegener's, but the lymphoma is much more destructive and can be differentiated histiologically.

Essential Investigations

Biopsy

This will not be diagnostic on its own but the presence of vasculitis and giant cells is highly suspicous of the disease.

C ANCA

Antineutrophil cytoplasmic antibody will be positive with a high titer *unless* the patient has already been treated with steroids or immunosuppressants.

Blood Tests

Complete blood count, ESR, CRP, creatinine, Rheumatoid factor.

Urine Analysis

In case of renal involvement.

Radiology

Chest radiograph, CT, and MRI scans of the diseased area.

Treatment

The aim of treatment is to prevent progression of the disease. High doses of steroids and azothioprine are the mainstay of treatment. Cyclophosphamide is also used. Immunotherapy (raising immunoglobulin levels) is beneficial to 30% of patients. Nasal symptoms can be controlled with saline inhalations (via spray or nebulizer) and trimethoprin cream may be helpful.

The ESR level (and sometimes the ANCA) is used to monitor the disease activity.

Sarcoidosis

Sarcoidosis is a systemic disease of unknown etiology. It commonly affects the nose. Deep granulomatous plaques form in the skin, giving a bulbous red tip to the nose (Fig 21-5). Nodules form on the nasal mucosa and destruction of the nasal bones to produce saddling may occur. The Kviem test is used to assist diagnosis (intradermal injection of extract of spleen from a known case of sarcoid followed by skin biopsy 6 weeks later). Investigations should include a chest radiograph, ESR, and serum calcium.

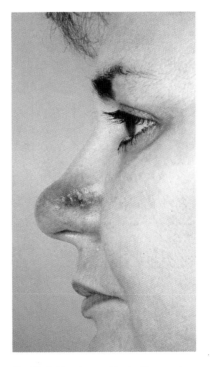

Fig 21-5 Nasal sarcoidosis. Deep granulomatous plaques in the skin give the characteristic bulbous red tip to the nose. (Photograph provided courtesy of Mr. R. Slack.)

Key Point:

The initial presentation of Wegener's granuloma may be to the Otolaryngology department with malaise, persistent nasal discharge, and granulation tissue in the nose.

The types of specific infections and nonspecific granulomas of the nose are summarized in Table 21-1.

Table 21-1. Specific Infections and Nonspecific Granulomas

Specific Infections	Nonspecific Granulomas
Fungal infections	Wegener's granuloma
AIDS	Sarcoidosis
Tuberculosis	
Syphilis	
Leprosy	

CHAPTER 22

Snoring and Obstructive Sleep Apnea

Snoring and obstructive sleep apnea (OSA) are due to partial or complete collapse of the pharyngeal airway during sleep. Airway patency is maintained by airway muscle tone and collapse results from any factors that narrow the airway or disturb the balance of these forces. These include nasal obstuction, excessive tonsillar tissue, or a narrow airway, which is usually due to obesity or an abnormal facial skeleton. Snoring and sleep apnea develop at sleep onset with the normal reduction in pharyngeal muscle tone that occurs at this time.

The sound of snoring is due to the partially obstructed pharyngeal airway and is due to turbulent airflow, which produces a vibrating air column. OSA ensues when the balance of pharyngeal forces leads to complete pharyngeal collapse. A mismatch between receptors in the chest wall and the lung causes an arousal from sleep and reopening of the airway.

Snoring and OSA represent extremes of a continuous spectrum of abnormality. Approximately 10% of adult males are severe snorers (termed heroic) and at least 0.3% of the adult male population have OSA, which occurs in all positions of sleep.

Heroic snoring causes daytime sleepiness and the individual is at risk while driving and occasionally from a partner driven to violence. However, unlike OSA, snoring is not associated with medical morbidity.

OSA is a serious condition that carries an increased risk of cardiovascular incident.

THE ASSESSMENT OF SNORING AND OSA

Medical and surgical therapies are available to treat snoring and OSA. The aim of treatment is to improve the airway patency by optimizing the balance of forces across the airway wall. The selection of the most appropriate therapy requires the following information:

1. Whether the snoring is present and is intrusive enough to warrant treatment.

2. The anatomical cause for the upper airway obstruction.

3. The presence and severity of any OSA.

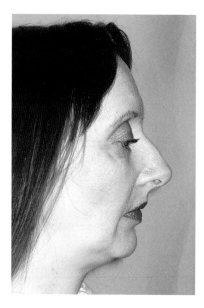

Fig 22-1 A retrognathia may be the cause of snoring.

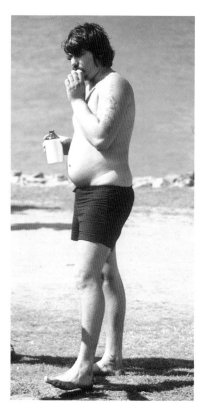

Fig 22-2 This individual has all of the risk factors for snoring. He is male, obese, and has a heavy alcohol intake. (Photograph provided courtesy of Dr. D. Babbs.)

History

It is helpful to interview the spouse with the patient. Questions are asked about the frequency and severity of the snoring, whether it occurs in all positions, and its relationship to alcohol intake.

A partner who is forced to sleep in a separate room is a useful marker of a substantial problem. Questions are also asked about excessive daytime sleepiness, restless sleep, and gaps in the breathing pattern.

Examination

Physical examination attempts to identify the anatomical cause for upper airway collapse. Look for obesity and abnormalities of the jaw (a small mandible crowds the retroglossal airway, Fig 22-1). An obese individual deposits fat around the pharynx and so narrows the upper airway (Fig 22-2). The nasal airway and pharynx is examined with rigid and flexible fiberoptic telescopes (Fig 22-3). The site of anatomical obstruction may be in the nose, at the level of the palate, at the tongue base, or at a combination of these 3 sites.

Radiological investigation (lateral cephalogram or CT) is occasionally used to identify masses impinging on the airway and to quantify retrognathia.

Sleep Study

All patients being considered for surgery for snoring or OSA should have a sleep study (Fig 22-4). This is to confirm and quantify the presence of snoring and or OSA.

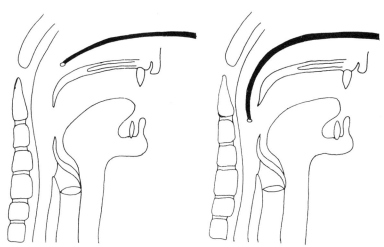

Fig 22-3 Diagram showing the principle of examination of the postnasal space with a flexible nasopharyngoscope.

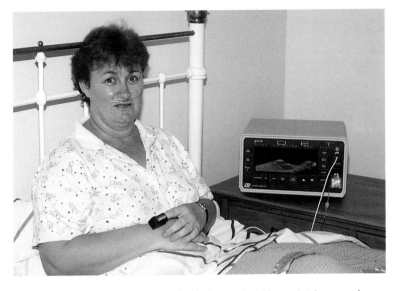

Fig 22-4 Sleep study is recommended before undertaking palatal surgery for snoring.

THE TREATMENT OF SNORING AND OSA

All patients should be advised to lose weight and cut down on excessive alcohol consumption where appropriate. Nasal obstruction should be treated either medically (eg, topical steroids) or surgically (eg, septoplasty). It is logical to do this first before embarking on more "adventurous" surgery.

In individuals with a retrognathic mandible, a dental prosthesis may be worn at night to keep the mandible forward and so enlarge the retroglossal airway. These devices attach to the teeth and are tolerated by some individuals.

Palatal Surgery

Uvulopalatopharyngoplasty (UPPP)

The principle of UPPP is to increase the oropharyngeal airway without jeopardizing the functions of the soft palate. If the patient's tonsils are present they are removed and then a small section of the soft palate including the uvula is resected, usually with a laser (Fig 22-5). At the end of the procedure, all the dimensions of the oropharyngeal airway have been increased (Fig 22-6). The postoperative management of UPPP patients is particularly important. Careful observation of the patient's airway is required and generous analgesia should be given.

In well-selected patients, UPPP works well and provides a permanent cure for snoring unless the patient becomes obese. The role of UPPP for individuals with OSA is less clear, being effective in approximately 50% of OSA patients. The OSA patients

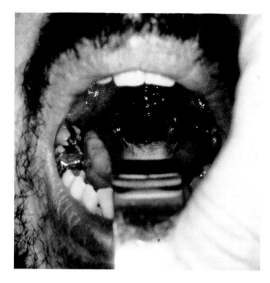

Fig 22-5 A crowded pharynx of the typical snorer—large tonsils and a long floppy soft palate.

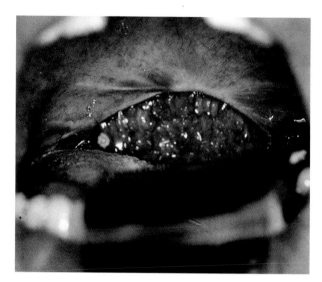

Fig 22-6 A UPPP operation removes excessive tissue and enlarges the velopalatine airway.

most likely to respond are those with airway obstruction at the level of the palate rather than the tongue base.

Laser-assisted Palatoplasty (LAUP)

This is a modification of the UPPP operation. It is often performed under local anesthesia with the patient sitting upright. Using a laser, vertical incisions are made through the palate on each side of the uvula. The uvula is shortened and reshaped (Fig 22-7).

Tonsillectomy Alone

In patients with huge obstructive tonsils, their removal alone may cure snoring and significantly reduce OSA if it is present (Fig 22-8).

Tracheostomy

This cures snoring and OSA but a hole in the neck has its own problems.

Continous Positive Airway Pressure (CPAP)

CPAP consists of a small mask connected to a pump that supplies positive pressure to the upper airway, thereby preventing collapse. It is not the most romantic device but it works for patients with OSA (Fig 22-9). OSA patients generally feel so terrible that they will comply with CPAP and indeed take it with them on holiday!

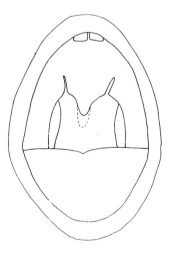

Fig 22-7 Diagram showing the LAUP procedure. Troughs are cut in each side of the soft palate and the uvula is shortened.

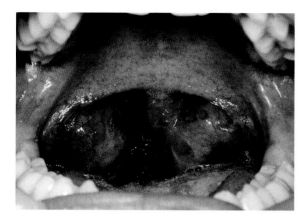

Fig 22-8 Huge obstructive tonsils may cause snoring and contribute to obstructive sleep apnea.

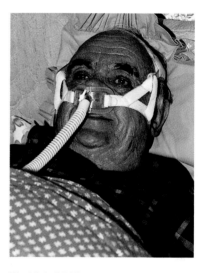

Fig 22-9 CPAP—continuous positive airway pressure—is the gold standard of treatment for obstructive sleep apnea. It's not a romantic device, however.

Key Points:

1. Snoring and obstructive sleep apnea (OSA) are due to partial or complete collapse of the pharyngeal airway during sleep.

2. Snoring and OSA represent extremes of a continuous spectrum of abnormality.

3. Heroic snorers are chronically tired and may die at the wheel or at the hands of their spouse!

4. OSA is associated with oxygen desaturation, pulmonary hypertension, and cardiac arrhythmias.

5. Weight loss and alcohol reduction are essential early measures in management of both OSA and snoring.

6. The aim of treatment is to improve the airway patency and may involve nasal and/or palatal surgery, or CPAP for OSA patients.

CHAPTER 23

Pituitary Disease

The management of pituitary disease requires a team approach. Overall responsibility lies with the endocrinologist. Otolaryngologists, neurosurgeons, and radiotherapists may participate in the treatment. Surgery is the most commonly used method for treating pituitary tumors. The indications for surgery are either to deal with the local effects of the tumor (eg, loss of vision) or to treat a systemic medical disorder such as acromegaly.

LOCAL EFFECTS

A tumor extending upward presses on the optic chiasma and may produce any type of visual field defect—the classic bitemporal hemianopia being occasionally demonstrable.

The contents of the cavernous sinus may be affected (cranial nerves III, IV, and VI). Raised intracranial pressure is rare and papilloedema is exceptional.

Downward extension into the sphenoid and postnasal space may present with CSF leak and recurrent meningitis.

SYSTEMIC EFFECTS

Acromegaly

The tumor secretes growth hormone and may be small (microadenoma) or replace most of the gland (Figs 23-1 and 23-2). High resolution CT scans and MRI can demonstrate microadenomas, and surgical removal leaving some normal gland behind is possible. Surgery is the most effective form of treatment for acromegaly.

Cushing's Disease

Cushing's can result from pituitary tumors that secrete ACTH, excessive steroid intake, an adrenal tumor, and ectopic ACTH-secreting tumors. The pituitary tumors are often microadenomas that are amenable to surgery with excellent results.

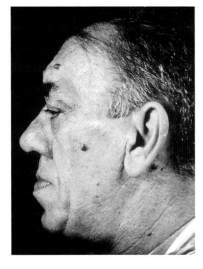

Fig 23-1 Acromegaly. Note the coarse features of the leonine facies, simian ridges, and protuberant lower jaw. The referral letter asked: "Does this patient have acromegaly or is he just ugly?"

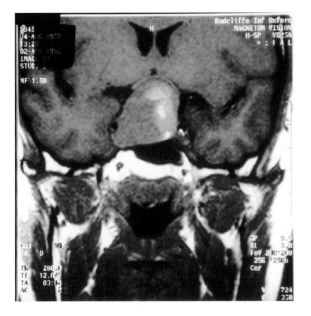

Fig 23-2 MRI showing a pituitary tumor. (Photograph provided courtesy of Dr. P. Anslow.)

Increased Prolactin Secretion

This can result from a tumor that secretes prolactin or from pressure effects in the region of the pituitary and hypothalamus. The condition presents with amenorrhea, infertility, and galactorrhea in women and gynacomastia in men.

Microdissection or medical treatment with bromocriptine is effective.

SURGICAL APPROACHES TO THE PITUITARY GLAND

The pituitary gland can be approached in 2 main ways:

1. *From below:* (trans-sphenoidal). This is the method of choice for excising the majority of tumors. An endoscopic approach to the sphenoid can be used or alternatively a transethmoid approach to the sphenoid can be employed. In the latter case a small external incision is made and the surgeon can obtain a binocular view by using the operating microscope.

2. *From above:* (craniotomy). If the tumor has significant upward extension then an approach from above is usually required, although, it can be combined with an endoscopic resection from below as well.

> **Key Point:**
>
> Any patient with progressive visual loss in whom the acuity cannot be corrected to 6/9 or better by refraction should be referred for neuro-ophthalmological assessment to exclude a compressive lesion, such as a pituitary tumor.

CHAPTER 24

Pediatric Rhinology

MANAGEMENT OF A NASAL MASS IN A CHILD

Many different entities may present as a nasal mass. It is important to remember that ethmoidal polyps are extremely rare under the age of 2 years. Preoperative radiological investigation is of the utmost importance. The mass can be aspirated to check for the presence of CSF before a biopsy is taken. If there is no connection with the cranial cavity, removal via the nose or a lateral rhinotomy is usually possible.

Table 24-1. Nasal Masses

Dermoids
Meningocoele
Nasal glioma
Lymphoma
Rhabdomyosarcoma
Nasopharyngeal carcinoma

Differential Diagnosis of a Nasal Mass in Childhood

Nasal masses may present in childhood and pose a challenging diagnostic problem (Table 24-1).

Nasal Dermoid Cysts

These occur in the midline and are due to entrapment of epithelial cells (Fig 24-1). A sinus may be present marked by a small dimple onto the skin. Occasionally, the sinus track may extend up to the dura so that a preoperative CT scan is essential.

Meningocoele

A meningocoele is a herniation of dura that includes CSF and brain tissue. It presents either as a soft tissue mass at the root of the nose or as an intranasal swelling looking like a polyp. CT scans are required to determine the extent of the meningocoele and the associated skull base defect.

Nasal Glioma

This is merely a solid mass of glial tissue that becomes entrapped outside the skull. The connection with the dura is usually lost and the cranium is intact. Most occur outside the nasal cavity and present as a lump on the nasal bridge, but some are entirely intranasal.

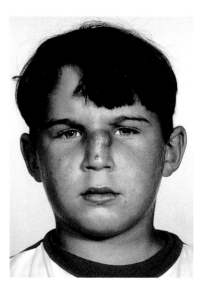

Fig 24-1 Midline nasal dermoid. This dermoid had no intracranial connection and was surgically removed from within the nose.

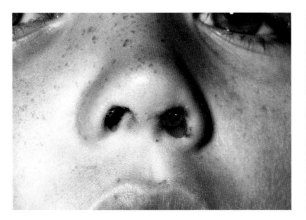

Fig 24-2 Unilateral nasal discharge in a child may indicate the presence of a foreign body. However, in this case, unilateral smelly discharge was treated for months as sinusitis. Eventually, the child was shown to have a rhabdomyosarcoma of the nasopharynx.

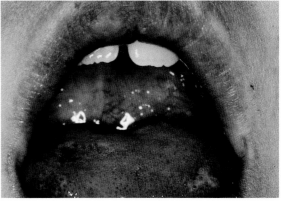

Fig 24-3 Same child shown in Fig 24-2 with a rhabdosarcoma of the nasopharynx. Note the soft palate is being pushed downward. On examination, the child sounded hyponasal because of the obstruction in the nasopharynx.

Lymphoma

This is the most common malignant tumor of childhood and can present as a mass arising from the back of the nose. Combination radiotherapy and chemotherapy now offer high cure rates.

Rhabdomyosarcomas

This is the second most common childhood malignancy, although it is rare in the nose and sinuses. The tumor can develop in many sites in the head and neck, including the sinuses, the nose, and the orbit (Figs 24-2 and 24-3). Treatment involves combinations of chemotherapy, radiotherapy, and surgery and should be undertaken in a pediatric oncology unit.

Nasopharyngeal Carcinoma

This carcinoma has a bimodal age distribution and does affect young people, particularly those of Chinese descent (p207).

Choanal Atresia

This is a bony (90%) or membranous (10%) occlusion at the back of the nose (posterior choanae). The atresia may be bilateral or unilateral. A newborn child is an obligate nasal breather, so complete bilateral choanal atresia is a fatal condition unless an oral airway is inserted. Often the baby exhibits cyclic cyanosis: Initially blue, the baby then cries with the result that the cyanosis is temporarily relieved.

Bilateral choanal atresia requires surgical intervention. The stenosis can usually be perforated with a probe and a silastic tube

Key Point:

In a child with unilateral nasal symptoms, exclude foreign bodies and tumor.

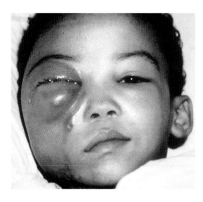

Fig 24-4 Child with acute ethmoiditis—a surgical emergency often requiring orbital decompression to save the vision.

inserted on both sides through the choanae. A CT will give details of the extent of atresia prior to surgery. Repeated dilations may lead to an adequate opening or the atretic plate may need to be drilled out as an elective procedure.

Unilateral choanal atresia may present late. The child or adult may have a unilateral nasal discharge or experience difficulty when the patent nostril is occluded during breast feeding.

SINUSITIS IN CHILDHOOD

The facial skeleton in a newborn infant is dominated by the ethmoid sinuses which make up 50% of the vertical dimension. Acute ethmoiditis develops rapidly and can have serious complications. Pus in the ethmoid sinus may erode through the lamina papyracea and lead to an orbital abscess.

The child presents with a history of pain around the eye (Fig 24-4). The symptoms and signs develop rapidly, and if the diagnosis is suspected, urgent hospital admission is required. Proptosis and periorbital edema are common. Limitation of eye movements and a reduction in visual acuity are sinister signs. If the condition does not respond rapidly to intravenous antibiotics, or if there is any loss of visual acuity, an urgent surgical exploration is required (see external ethmoidectomy p121).

Key Point:

The ethmoid sinus is the dominant sinus in children. Ethmoiditis frequently presents with orbital complications.

FOREIGN BODIES IN THE NOSE

Beads, pieces of rubber, paper, and all sorts of oddments are frequently inserted into the nostril by children. They may not be detected initially, but present with a unilateral purulent discharge. A good way of inspecting the nasal cavity in a child is to use the speculum of a fiberoptic auriscope (see Fig 11-10). This can be gently inserted without causing undue distress. If the child is cooperative, a foreign body in the anterior part of the nose can be removed by passing a probe under it and tipping it forward into the front of the nose. Frequently, a general anesthetic is required to allow removal of the object.

Key Point:

Unilateral, offensive, purulent nasal discharge in a child is usually due to foreign body.

NASAL TRAUMA IN CHILDHOOD

The child's nose is less prominent and more cartilaginous than its adult counterpart. It is thus able to withstand the many facial injuries sustained by children. Be mindful of the possibility of nonaccidental injury (Fig 24-5). Injuries (surgery included!) may interfere with the growth centers in the nose with resultant cosmetic deformities in later life (see Fig 17-4).

Surgical correction of childhood nasal deformity should be conservative. Cartilage may be repositioned but not resected. In many circumstances, it may be better to delay surgery until the nose has reached adult proportions.

RESPIRATORY OBSTRUCTION IN CHILDHOOD

Many children snore and a small proportion of these children have sleep apnea. This is usually due to enlarged tonsils and occasionally to enlarged adenoids (Fig 24-6). Obstructive apnea occurs when the tonsils totally block the airway so that no air enters despite strenuous respiratory efforts (sternal and intercostal recession can be seen). The low arterial oxygen then stimulates the respiratory center sufficiently to produce a massive inspiratory effort, which sucks the tonsils out of the way. The apnea then ends.

Children with respiratory obstruction during sleep do not grow as fast as their peers (decreased growth hormone secretion), and may have bedwetting and behavioral problems.

Severe snoring and obstructive apnea may lead to arrhythmias and right ventricular hypertrophy. Tonsillectomy and/or adenoidectomy cures the problem. In children with severe obstruction it is wise to obtain a chest radiograph and an ECG. The anesthetist should be informed in good time.

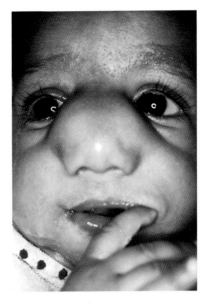

Fig 24-5 Nonaccidental injury. This grotesque injury was not accidental. This diagnosis could easily have been overlooked.

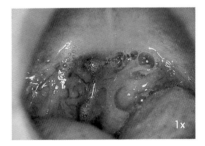

Fig 24-6 Enlarged tonsils causing snoring and obstructive sleep apnea.

Key Points:

1. Enlarged tonsils and adenoids may cause snoring and sleep apnea in childhood.

2. Small stature, bedwetting, and behavioral problems may be clues to sleep problems in children.

CHAPTER 25

Cosmetic Facial Plastic Surgery

Patients can become greatly concerned about their facial appearance and identification of a cosmetic problem and its surgical correction can be both challenging and satisfying.

RHINOPLASTY

The appearance and function of the nose are closely related. Some patients may be reluctant to discuss cosmetic concerns. It is most important to encourage an open and frank discussion. Patients should be helped to point out their perceived problems and then be given a realistic appraisal of what cosmetic facial surgery can achieve. Patients who cannot explain what it is they do not like about their nose, or who have unrealistic expectations, should not have an operation.

Abnormalities in the shape of the nose may be due to cartilaginous and/or bony defects. Some common abnormalities are shown in Figs 25-1 and 25-2.

The basic requirements of rhinoplasty are that the surgery should restore normal function to the nose and the appearance should be improved so that the nose harmonizes with the rest of the face.

A deviated septum often occurs with a cosmetic deformity, so the standard operation is termed a septo-rhinoplasty. A closed septo-rhinoplasty is performed through incisions made within the nasal vestibule. An open approach septo-rhinoplasty utilizes a tiny butterfly incision across the columella. In both methods, access is provided to the alar cartilages, nasal dorsum, and septum. Abnormalities in any one or all of these areas can then be corrected.

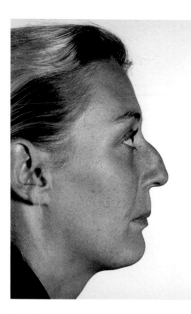

Fig 25-1 A dorsal "hump" arises from the nasal bones and cartilages.

Key Points:

1. A successful rhinoplasty should restore the normal structure and function of a nose. The reconstructed nose should harmonize with the rest of the face.

2. The rhinoplasty surgeon can enhance the patient's beauty in small increments only.

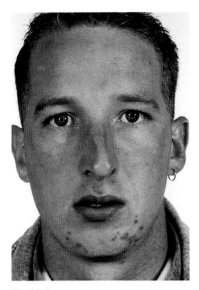
Fig 25-2a

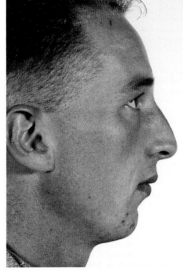
Fig 25-2b

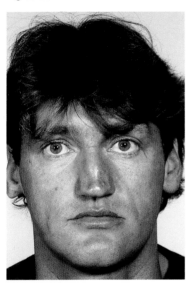
Fig 25-2c

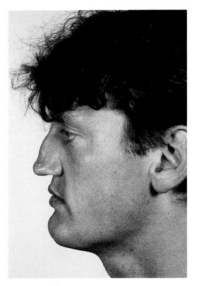
Fig 25-2d

Fig 25-2 The deviated nose.

MENTOPLASTY

The nose should not be considered in isolation. A retousse chin will make the nose appear large. Augmenting the chin will greatly improve the proportion of the face and may complement a rhinoplasty.

Projection of the chin can be increased with a silastic implant or by bone advancement.

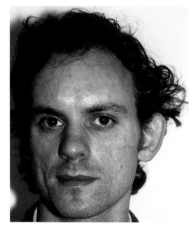 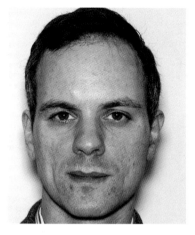

Fig 25-3 Pinnaplasty. This patient was on a waiting list for surgery from childhood.

Fig 25-4 Post-pinnaplasty (see Fig 25-3). The patient also demonstrates the esthetic merits of a hair cut!

OTOPLASTY

Prominent ears (Figs 25-3 and 25-4) are best corrected before a child starts school. The usual deformity results from failure to develop an antihelical fold. The aim of surgery is to create a new natural-looking fold and various techniques exist to "pin back" the protruding ears.

BLEPHAROPLASTY

Aging may result in redundant skin and fat pads in the upper and lower eyelids. A blepharoplasty is an operation in which excess skin and fat are removed from the eyelids (Figs 25-5 and 25-6).

FACELIFT

With increasing age, the elasticity of the skin is lost. This process is accelerated by sun exposure. In the facelift operation, incisions are made in the hair line and the excess skin is pulled up and trimmed off. Endoscopic techniques are now used for some facelifts, although not all patients are suitable.

LASER RESURFACING

Laser technology now allows the skin collagen to be reorganized and in effect tightened up. The procedure can be performed in the office under local anesthetic. "Crow's feet" and wrinkles can be removed.

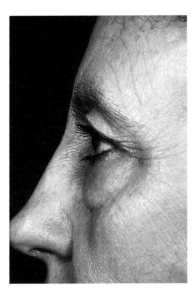 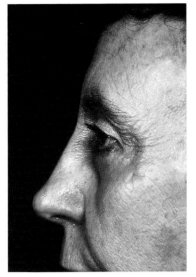

Fig 25-5 Preblepharoplasty. Note the "bags" under the lower eyelid.

Fig 25-6 Same patient shown in Fig 25-5 following blepharoplasty.

INJECTION OF BOTULINUM TOXIN

This is another method for removing wrinkles. A small dose of the toxin is injected and the wrinkle disappears as the underlying muscle is weakened. The effect of the toxin lasts for a few weeks, when another injection can be given. Botulinum toxin is also used in the treatment of various dystonias, including spasmodic dystonia, and in the treatment of facial paralysis.

HAIR TRANSPLANTS

Almost every patient with male pattern baldness can be helped by some form of surgical hair restoration if they so wish.

PART THREE

The Larynx, Head and Neck

CHAPTER 26

Clinical Anatomy and Physiology

....

THE ORAL CAVITY AND PHARYNX

Many ENT diseases arise in this area and familiarity with the anatomy and physiology is important. The oral cavity contains the upper and lower dentition, the tongue and floor of the mouth, the hard palate, and the openings of the major salivary glands (Figs 26-1 and 26-2). The area between the teeth and the cheeks (bucco-alveolar sulcus) is easily overlooked. The anterior border of the tonsil is known as the anterior pillar of the fauces and marks the start of the pharynx itself.

The tongue may be divided into an anterior two thirds and a posterior one third. The anterior two thirds comprises a dorsum, lateral borders and ventral surface. The posterior one third of the tongue is continuous posteriorly with the epiglottis; between these two areas lie two small depressions known as valleculae which may be the site of food impaction.

The floor of the mouth is supported by the mylohyoid muscles, which stretch between the rami of mandible like a hammock and are joined in the midline.

The oral cavity is lined by stratified squamous epithelium and it contains many small salivary glands ('minor' salivary glands). The blood supply is from branches of the external carotid artery. The lymphatic drainage is to ipsilateral submental and sub-mandibular lymph nodes but the anterior floor of mouth and base of tongue have considerable "crossover" and drain to both sides of the neck.

The *sensory nerve* supply of the tongue is from the lingual nerve (Trigeminal-V) in the anterior two thirds and Glossopharyngeal nerve (IX) posteriorly. The *motor supply* is from the hypoglossal nerve (XII). The *blood supply* is mainly from the lingual artery which is a direct branch of the external carotid artery.

THE TONSILS

This normally refers to the palatine tonsils which lie adjacent to the posterior one third of the tongue but it should be remembered that there is a complete ring of lymphoid tissue (Waldeyer's ring) which comprises the adenoids (pharyngeal tonsils) (p), the palatine tonsils,

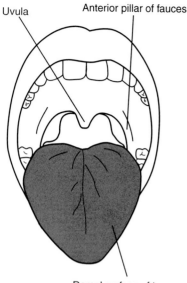

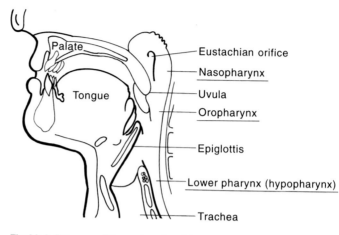

Fig 26-2 Diagram of the oral cavity with tongue touching hard palate and illustrating openings of submandibular ducts.

Fig 26-1 Diagrammatic representation of the oral cavity with tongue protruded.

and the lingual and pharyngeal tonsils. The latter are situated laterally on the posterior pharyngeal wall and are sometimes known as the lateral pharyngeal bands.

Immunological Functions

The palatine tonsils are placed at the entry of the food and air passages and are constantly exposed to new antigens, unlike most of the lymphoid tissue in the body. They are part of the mucosal associated lymphoid tissues (MALT) and probably process antigen and present it to T helper (TH) cells and B cells. Although the majority of MALT cells produce IgA, the tonsillar tissue mainly produces IgG; IgA represents only about 35 percent of its secretions. IgD is also seen but represents less than 5 percent of secretions. These immunoglobulins pass directly out into the pharyngeal secretions and their output is enhanced in the presence of inflammation.

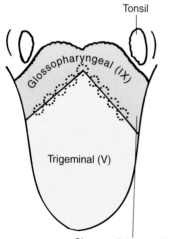

Fig 26-3 Dorsum of tongue showing the V-shaped partition between the anterior two thirds and the posterior one third, and the circumvallate papillae at the junction and the sensory nerve supply to the different parts.

TASTE

The taste buds are made up of four different cell types, which are found in the lingual epithelium. Microvilli project from the upper surface of these cells and are in contact with fluids in the mouth. In man, these cells lie in the mucosa of the oral cavity and pharynx but are also concentrated in the fungiform papillae in the anterior tongue and the circumvallate papillae, which lie in an inverted V-shape at the junction of the anterior two thirds and posterior one third of the dorsum of the tongue (Fig. 26-3).

The taste sensations are transmitted to the tractus solitarius in the brain stem via 2 different routes:

Anterior Two-Thirds Tongue

Afferent fibers travel from the tongue in the chorda tympani nerve which joins the facial nerve (VII) in the middle ear and passes into the posterior cranial fossa via the internal auditory meatus.

Posterior One-Third Tongue

Fibers pass via the glossopharyngeal nerve (IX) and enter the posterior fossa via the jugular foramen.

There are only four fundamental tastes: sweet, sour, bitter and salt. Much of what we perceive as taste is really olfaction (p89) and patients who are anosmic often think they have lost their sense of taste and smell together. Accurate testing is very difficult due to the problems of standardizing stimuli.

> **Key Point:**
> Most of taste is actually due to the sense of smell.

SWALLOWING

This is a reflex which is mediated via *afferent* fibers passing to the medulla oblongata through the second division of the trigeminal (V), the glossopharyngeal (IX), and vagus (X) nerves. The *efferent* pathway is from the nucleus ambiguus and is mediated via the glossopharyngeal (IX), vagus (X), and hypoglossal (XII) nerves.

Oral Phase

This comes first and involves the preparation of a food bolus in the oral cavity using teeth, tongue, and muscles of mastication. This is under voluntary control.

Reflex Phase

This phase comes next and is initiated by displacement of the food bolus posteriorly by elevation of the tongue. Entry of the bolus into the oropharynx initiates the swallow and includes:

1. Inhibition of respiration and closure of the nasopharynx by elevation of the soft palate.

2. Elevation of the larynx under the tongue base.

3. Decrease of pressure in the lower pharynx and passage of the food bolus past the larynx into the 2 pyriform fossae towards the esophageal inlet by a series of contractions of the pharyngeal constrictor muscles.

4. Relaxation of the cricopharyngeus muscle and peristalsis of the esophageal musculature and transport of the bolus through to the stomach.

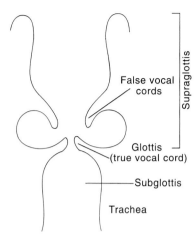

Fig 26-4 Schematic vertical section through the larynx demonstrating the main anatomical and clinical subdivisions.

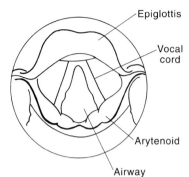

Fig 26-5 A diagram of the larynx as seen during mirror laryngoscopy.

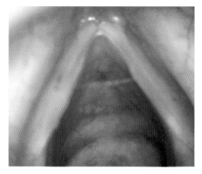

Fig 26-6 A normal larynx as seen during fiberoptic laryngoscopy.

This process is sufficient to propel a food bolus even against the effects of gravity—thus enabling people to drink pints of beer while upside down!

THE LARYNX

The larynx is a protective sphincter at the inlet of the tracheo-bronchial tree and is also responsible for the generation of sound. It has a mainly cartilaginous framework consisting of the hyoid bone above, the thyroid cartilage and cricoid cartilage below, and the arytenoid cartilages posteriorly. The cricoid cartilage is the only complete ring of cartilage in the entire airway. The larynx is situated in the anterior neck and its posterior wall is the same as the anterior wall of the pharynx. The epiglottis projects superiorly from the front of the larynx and acts like the lid of a box.

By convention the larynx is divided into supraglottis, glottis, and subglottis. The true vocal cords (ie, glottis) are white and contain the vocal ligaments which are at the medial end of the thyro-arytenoid muscles. Above the muscles are two medial projections known as the false cords (Fig 26-4).

The true vocal cords meet anteriorly near to the thyroid prominence (Adam's apple). Posteriorly they are separate and each is attached to one arytenoid cartilage. This gives a V-shape in appearance (Figs 26-5 and 26-6).

The arytenoid cartilages articulate with the posterior part of the cricoid cartilage just below the glottis. The thyroid cartilage is also V-shaped and is open posteriorly.

Sensory Nerve Supply

The sensory nerve supply to the larynx above the vocal cords is from the *superior laryngeal nerve*. Below the vocal cords it is from the *recurrent laryngeal nerve*. Both of these nerves are branches of the vagus (X).

Motor Nerve Supply

The movements of the vocal cords and the intrinsic muscles of the larynx are controlled by the recurrent laryngeal nerve which is a branch of the vagus (X). The exception is the cricothyroid muscle, which is supplied by the superior laryngeal nerve.

Key Point:

1. Only the posterior cricoarytenoid muscles abduct the cords; all other intrinsic laryngeal muscles adduct the cords.

2. These muscles are supplied by the recurrent laryngeal nerves which, if damaged, may therefore produce closure of the airway.

Lymphatics

The lymphatic drainage is different above and below the glottis, which acts as a watershed (ie, just like the innervation). The lymphatic drainage of the supraglottis is to the upper deep cervical nodes whereas that of the subglottis is to nodes along the internal jugular vein and also to peritracheal and mediastinal nodes.

Voice Production

The lungs, diaphragm, and abdomen provide a source of air. The larynx channels this into a column of high-speed vibrating air which is then converted into intelligible speech by the remainder of the vocal tract—ie, the pharynx, tongue, lips, resonating chambers of the head, etc.

In brief, the larynx functions by closing the vocal cords against the air pressure from below, which is created by exhalation. This causes a rise in subglottic pressure, which forces the cords apart slightly for an instant. The subglottic pressure is thus reduced for a moment and the cords come together again (the Bernoulli effect). This occurs in rapid sequence to produce a vibrating stream of air emanating from the lungs.

Pitch is controlled by the frequency of the vocal cord vibrations, which in turn are determined by the thickness, length, and tension of the cords. Intensity is governed by air pressure and the amplitude of vibrations.

Modern research using stroboscopy has shown the importance of the mucosal wave across the surface of the vocal fold and this has led to changes in our understanding of laryngeal surgery.

Key Points:

1. The vocal ligament itself has no lymphatic drainage, hence tumours confined to the vocal ligament do not metastasize.

2. The glottis demarcates the neurovascular supply to the larynx. Above the cords, sensory innervation is from the superior laryngeal nerve. Below the cords, it is from the recurrent laryngeal nerve.

3. All the intrinsic muscles of the larynx are supplied by the recurrent laryngeal nerve with the exception of the cricothyroid muscle.

THE NECK

The neck can be divided into triangles: the sternomastoid muscle separates the posterior triangle from the anterior triangle. The posterior triangle extends backward to the anterior border of trapezius and inferiorly to the clavicle. The anterior triangle extends to

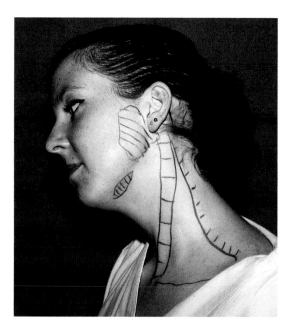

Fig 26-7 Surface markings of the parotid and submandibular glands. The anterior border of the sternomastoid muscle is also identified as is the anterior rim of the trapezius muscle and the level of the clavicle.

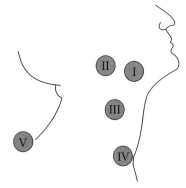

Fig 26-8 Scheme of main lymph node groups in the neck: I submandibular; II, III, IV—upper, middle and lower deep cervical; V—posterior triangle.

the midline and the upper part may be subdivided into the submandibular triangle (above the digastric muscle) and submental triangle (between the anterior bellies of the digastric) (Fig 26-7).

The *lymphatic drainage* of the head and neck is of great clinical significance. While a small chain of nodes exists in the upper neck (submental, submandibular, preauricular, occipital), the most important chain is the deep cervical nodes, which run adjacent to the internal jugular vein. They are usually divided into four regions: the jugulodigastric ("tonsillar node"), which is known as level II and the upper, middle, and lower deep cervical nodes (Fig. 26-8), which are classified as levels I, III, and IV in that order. When enlarged, they can be palpated along the anterior border of the sternomastoid muscle but they also lie underneath this muscle and their true size when enlarged can be very difficult to determine clinically.

THE SALIVARY GLANDS

Humans produce approximately 600 ml of saliva each day. The main salivary glands are pairs of structures parotid, submandibular, and sublingual. These are known as the major glands.

The parotid gland is composed almost entirely of serous acini. The submandibular is a mixture of serous and mucinous acini (mainly serous), and the sublingual consists mainly of mucinous acini. There are also thousands of small collections of salivary tissue throughout the upper aerodigestive tract known as the minor salivary glands.

Saliva contains two enzymes—*ptyalin* which comes from the major salivary glands and is an amylase and *lingual lipase.* It also contains mucin which is a glycoprotein and acts as a lubricant fluid; immunogloblins including IgA, IgG, and IgD are also found. Saliva performs many functions including moistening, dissolving some molecules, facilitating speech articulation, and keeping the mouth clean by washing away bacteria around the teeth.

Secretion of Saliva

The secretion of saliva is controlled by the *parasympathetic secreto-motor fibers* that synapse in ganglia near their end organ as follows:

1. *Parotid gland* via the glossopharyngeal nerve (IX). The tympanic branch sends fibers via the lesser superficial petrosal nerve to the otic ganglion. The postganglionic fibers then "hitchhike" with the auriculotemporal nerve, which is a branch of the trigeminal (V).

2. *Submandibular gland* via the facial nerve (VII). The fibers pass to the submandibular ganglion in the chorda tympani to the lingual nerve.

3. *Sublingual gland* via the facial nerve (VII). This receives its secretomotor supply in the same fashion as the submandibular gland.

The postganglionic fibers which enter the glands cause local release of acetylcholine or vasoactive intestinal peptide (VIP), which is a cotransmitter. This neurosecretion is initiated by the presence of fluid in the mouth or stomach. It can also be stimulated by the sight, smell, or thought of food—as in Pavlov's original experiments on the conditioning of dogs.

THE THYROID GLAND

Anatomy

The thyroid is an endocrine gland which secretes tri-iodothyronine—T3, tetra-iodothyronine—T4/thyroxine and calcitonin. It lies in the lower neck and weighs 20–30 g; it consists of 2 lateral lobes connected by a narrow midline isthmus, which overlies the 2nd–4th tracheal rings. It receives arterial blood from the superior thyroid artery—a branch of the external carotid—and the inferior thyroid artery, which is a branch of the thyrocervical trunk. The posterior border is related to the esophagus, and the recurrent laryngeal nerves lie in the groove between the trachea and esophagus, covered by the thyroid gland. These nerves are closely related to the inferior thyroid arteries. The gland consists of two types of secretory cells: *follicles*, which are lined with epithelium and contain colloid, and *parafollicular cells,* which secrete calcitonin.

Function

The thyroid gland functions by trapping iodide from the blood which is coupled with tyrosine to form T3 and T4. The circulating levels of thyroid hormones are monitored by the hypothalamus-pituitary axis and *thyroid stimulating hormone* (TSH) is secreted from the anterior pituitary as required. This is a classical biological feedback mechanism. The hormones themselves are stored as colloid within the follicles. The height of the epithelial cells in the follicles is controlled by TSH secretion. The parafollicular cells are of neural crest origin and are involved in calcium homeostasis.

Embryology

The gland develops in the floor of the pharynx from a thickening that forms the thyroglossal duct. This elongates and descends early in fetal development, prior to ossification of the hyoid bone, to reach its eventual site in the lower neck by the third fetal month. The duct then breaks up but a small pit on the dorsum of the posterior third of the tongue—the foramen caecum—remains to mark the origin of the duct. Abnormal thyroid tissue may be seen anywhere along the track of the thyroglossal duct but is almost always midline (p45).

THE PARATHYROIDS

Anatomy

The superior and inferior parathyroids are small (0.5 cm) glands derived from the third and fourth pharyngeal pouches, respectively, and are usually attached to the posterior part of the thyroid gland. Their exact position is very variable although the superior glands are about the size of a small pea and are related to the vascular pedicle on the posterosuperior part of the thyroid lobes. The inferior pair of parathyroids are more variable in position and may occasionally be found in the superior mediastinum.

Function

The parathyroid glands secrete *parathormone*, which maintains calcium and phosphorus homeostasis via a complex interaction with the gastrointestinal tract, skeletal system, kidneys, and vitamin D. Loss of parathyroid tissue (eg, after laryngectomy) leads to hypocalcaemia and *tetanic muscle spasm*.

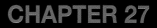

CHAPTER 27

Examination of the Head and Neck

THE ORAL CAVITY

Clinical examination requires a bright light and a tongue depressor—a right-angled metal tongue depressor is very useful for this. ENT surgeons customarily use a reflecting mirror on the head or a headband-mounted fiberoptic light source, which permits use of both hands to move the tongue and hold instruments. Always examine the bucco-alveolar sulcus and the floor of the mouth. Examination without a tongue depressor is inadequate (Figs 27-1, 27-2, & 27-3). Generalized diseases may often be identified from examination of the oral cavity—for example, the tongue fasciculation of motor neurone disease, the brown mucosal pigmentation of Addison's disease, the macroglossia of acromegaly, hypoglossal nerve palsy (Fig 27-4), or tongue-tie (Fig 27-5).

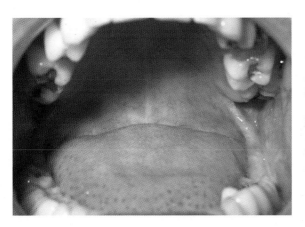

Fig 27-1 Examination of mouth without a tongue depressor rarely reveals much information except the presence or absence of the tongue!

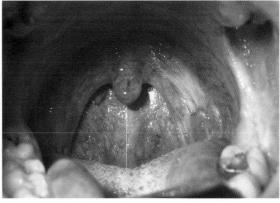

Fig 27-2 Examination of same patient with tongue depressor in place.

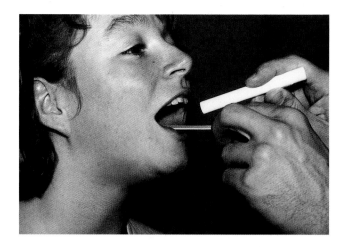

Fig 27-3 Examination of the mouth in a cooperative adult with a pen torch and wooden tongue depressor.

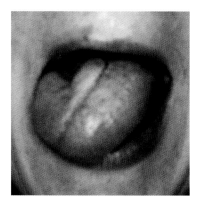

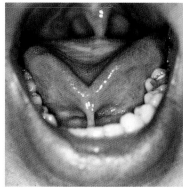

Fig 27-4 A case of hypoglossal nerve palsy (XII). Note that the tongue always deviates to the side of the palsy.

Fig 27-5 A case of a short lingual frenulum (tongue tie).

THE LARYNX, PHARYNX, AND NASOPHARYNX

Indirect Laryngoscopy (Fig 27-6)

This allows visualization of the larynx down to the level of the vocal cords. The tongue is protruded and held by the examiner while a warm mirror (Fig 27-7) is placed on the posterior soft palate. In experienced hands it can be done rapidly and usually without any anesthetic. It permits assessment of cord mobility as well as identification of mass lesions. The upper part of the pharynx and posterior part of the tongue are also seen with this technique. In some patients with a pronounced gag reflex, the procedure may be facilitated by use of a local anaesthetic spray such as lignocaine. This old fashioned technique is quick but does not allow demonstration of abnormalities to the patient.

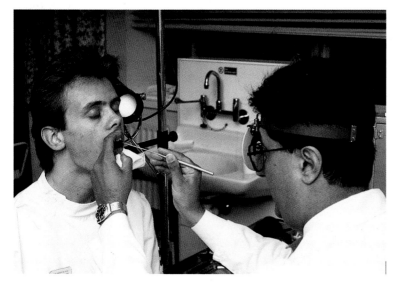

Fig 27-6 Mirror examination of the larynx in a cooperative patient.

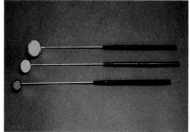

Fig 27-7 A set of laryngeal mirrors as used for indirect laryngoscopy. These mirrors have to be warmed before insertion into the mouth.

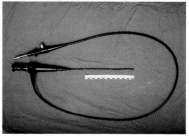

Fig 27-8 Equipment for fiberoptic examination of the pharynx and larynx.

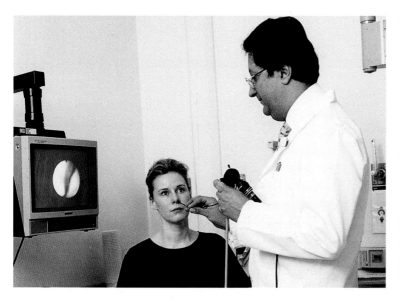

Fig 27-9 Demonstration of fiberoptic assessment of the larynx with the nasendoscope in outpatients under local anaesthesia with the use of a video camera.

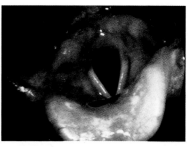

Fig 27-10 Normal larynx photographed using a nasendoscope (see also Figs 30-1 and 30-2).

Fiberoptic Laryngoscopy

This may be performed with a rigid or flexible endoscope (Fig 27-8) and provides a clear view of all the structures involved. The fiberoptic nasendoscope is passed through the nose under topical anesthesia (with cocaine) and the entire nasopharynx and larynx can be seen and demonstrated to others. It also permits photography for documentation of specific lesions. (Figs 27-9, 27-10, and

Key Point:

Thorough inspection of the larynx is essential in every hoarse patient.

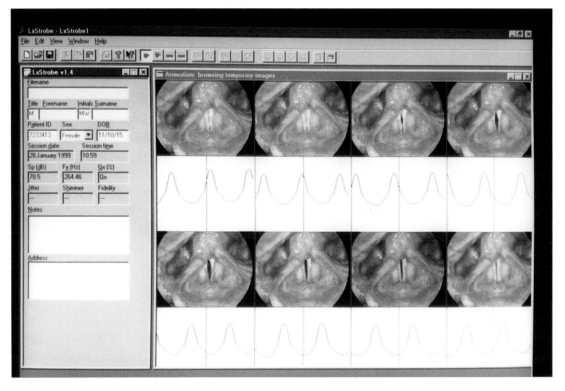

Fig 27-11 Photographic recording of laryngeal movements using a stroboscope (see also Voice Analysis, Chapter 30).

27-11). Camera-aided fiberoptic laryngoscopy is the ideal technique for laryngeal examination.

THE NECK

Expose the whole neck and inspect the neck from in front. Then stand behind the patient and flex the chin downward slightly to remove undue tension in the sternohyoid muscles and the platysma. Palpate the neck with the pulps of the fingers, not the tips (Fig 27-12). Palpate the deep chain of lymph nodes along the course of the interior jugular vein and deep to the belly of

Key Points:

1. An enlarged neck node is often much bigger than it appears on palpation.

2. When examining for a lump in the neck it is helpful to ask the patient to locate it first.

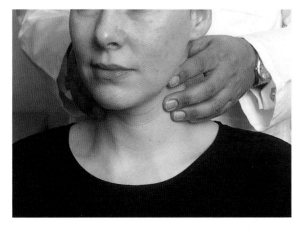

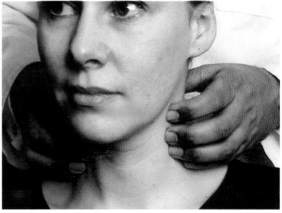

Fig 27-12 Examination of the neck. Always stand behind the patient and use the pulps not the tips of the fingers. Keep the neck slightly flexed.

Fig 27-13 Examination of the neck using the tips of the fingers. This is the wrong method.

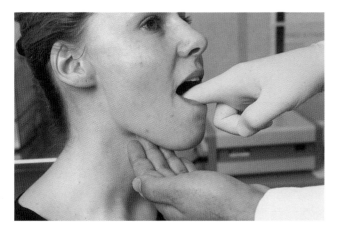

Fig 27-14 Bimanual examination of the submandibular gland with a gloved finger inserted intraorally.

the sternomastoid muscle and then the superficial chain around the upper neck. Check for normal laryngeal mobility and movement of any masses on swallowing and on tongue protrusion.

THE SALIVARY GLANDS

Examine the area around the gland that appears to be affected and compare it with the other side. Always inspect the opening of the salivary ducts and examine regional nerves. This means the facial nerve for parotid lesions and the hypoglossal and lingual nerves for submandibular lesions. The gland should also be palpated bimanually with a gloved finger inside the mouth (Fig 27-13 and 27-14). Do not let the patient open the mouth too wide as the surrounding muscles become tense and interfere with palpation.

Key Point:

Never examine the parotid without testing the facial nerve.

The key points in the history and examination are summarized in Table 27-1.

Table 27-1. ENT: History Taking and Examination

Ear	Nose	Throat
	History	
Earache, irritation	Obstruction	Hoarseness
Deafness	Rhinorrhoea /postnasal drip	Dysphagia
Discharge	Allergy/hay fever	Stridor
Tinnitus	Facial pain	Lump in the neck
Vertigo	Epistaxis	
	Sense of smell	Sleep disturbance
	Appearance	
Children: Speech/language		
	Past History	
Barotrauma	Trauma	Cigarette smoking
Acoustic trauma	Medications	Alcohol
Head injury	prescribed	
Ototoxics	nonprescribed	
Family history	Previous surgery	Previous surgery
Previous ear surgery		
	Examination	
Pinna	Shape	Mouth and tongue
Mastoid	Septum	(palates, gums, teeth, tonsils)
Ear canal	Turbinates	Neck swelling
Ear drum (esp.attic)	Mucopus?	Larynx—ENT
Tuning forks	Airway	
Conversational test	Facial tenderness	
Nystagmus	Facial sensation	
Facial nerve	Facial swelling	

CHAPTER 28

Investigation of Head and Neck Diseases

THE NECK

CT Scanning

CT scanning has replaced tomography as the investigation of choice for many disorders and shows bone erosion and encroachment onto the great vessels of the neck by tumors (Fig 28-1). Its lack of sophistication in showing soft tissue detail is a drawback.

MRI Scanning

The greater soft tissue definition of MRI scanning, which can be coupled with paramagnetic agents, means that this is now the investigation of choice in most neck diseases. It is an adjunct in the staging of carcinoma of the head and neck as it has a high success rate in identifying lymphatic enlargement but cannot differentiate true metastatic disease from reactive nodal enlargement. Accordingly, MRI scanning can lead to a high level of false positives in the neck.

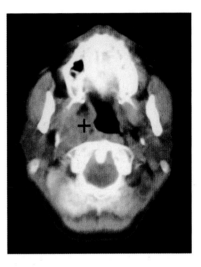

Fig 28-1 A CT scan showing gross obstruction of the pharynx on the right side (marked by +).

SWALLOWING

Barium Swallow

Swallowing has traditionally been assessed by very simple methods such as the barium swallow. ENT surgeons have in the past supplemented the simple barium liquid studies with a solid object such as a biscuit or marshmallow coated with dye (Figs 28-2 and 28-3).

Video Fluoroscopy and High-Speed Cine Recordings

Video fluoroscopy and high speed cine recordings allow the evaluation of the oral and pharyngeal phases in much more detail. Modified barium studies using barium-coated food such as biscuits are also valuable in this regard.

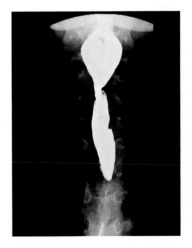

Fig 28-2 A-P and lateral view of a stricture in the postcricoid region and the typical "shouldered" appearance of a malignancy.

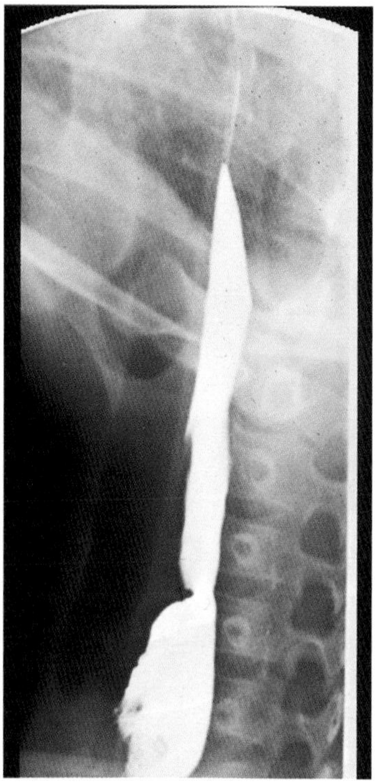

Manometric Analysis and pH Measurements

Manometric analysis and pH measurements are also used in specialized units to investigate gastroesophageal reflux; these can be coupled with simultaneous fluoroscopy.

THE LARYNX

Plain Lateral X Rays of the Neck

Plain lateral X rays of the neck can give a little information—especially about the airway and soft tissue abnormalities. The depth of the prevertebral soft tissue shadow can be a useful guide to the presence of disease in the hypopharynx (Fig 28-4). They can also give information about infection—eg, if there is air in the soft tissues; or they occasionally allow visualization of a foreign body.

CT Scanning

CT scanning is the modern way of imaging the larynx and has superceded tomography. It is particularly good at demonstrating the size and local extent of malignant disease (Fig 28-5).

Magnetic Resonance Imaging (MRI)

Magnetic resonance imaging is being used increasingly often and represents another new and important option. It can be used to assess local spread of tumors (Fig 28-6).

THE ORAL CAVITY

Orthopantomogram (OPT)

The OPT is a special radiological view that displays both upper and lower jaws and all the dentition on one X-ray plate (Fig 28-7). It is helpful if searching for bone erosion or peridontal infection.

Intraoral Dental Views

Intraoral dental views are helpful especially when identifying salivary calculi (Fig 28-8) (see also sialography).

Voice Analysis

Several techniques are available for the measurement of voice including electrolaryngography and electromyography of the laryngeal muscles. The most useful is videostroboscopy, which can

Fig 28-3 A-P and lateral view of a stricture in the postcricoid region and the typical "shouldered" appearance of a malignancy.

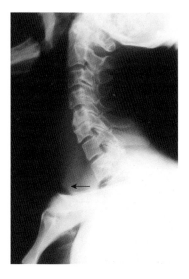

Fig 28-4 Gross enlargement of the prevertebral soft tissue shadow in a case of carcinoma of the hypopharynx (arrowed).

be undertaken as an outpatient technique with topical anesthesia. This utilizes a rigid nasendoscope coupled to a video camera and a stroboscopic light which flashes on and off at the same speed as the object being viewed. This "freezes" the image and enables the surgeon to identify the rhythm of the glottic movements and demonstrate this on a television screen to the patient and speech therapist. The use of digital cameras has allowed the laryngeal image to be captured and analyzed on almost any suitable personal computer. This technique has allowed much more sensitive assessment of the mucosal waveform of the glottis (Figs 27-11 and 28-9).

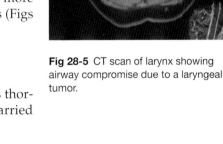

Fig 28-5 CT scan of larynx showing airway compromise due to a laryngeal tumor.

Direct Laryngoscopy and Microlaryngoscopy

Examination under general anesthesia (EUA). This permits thorough examination of the larynx and biopsy, and may be carried

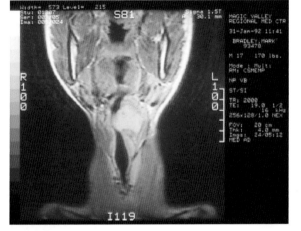

Fig 28-6 MRI of a laryngeal tumor with airway obstruction (coronal section).

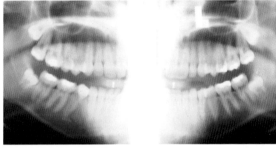

Fig 28-7 A normal orthopantomogram in a young adult female.

out with the aid of the operating microscope (microlaryngoscopy), which facilitates the photographic documentation of pathology. It is increasingly being replaced by fiberoptic examination (see above) but remains the mainstay of assessment in cases of suspected cancer. Microlaryngoscopy also permits the specific treatment of certain disorders such as polyps (p193). (see Fig 27-11)

NECK DISEASE

Angiography or Digital Subtraction Vascular Imaging

This is essential if a vascular lesion is suspected and also has a therapeutic role by facilitating embolization.

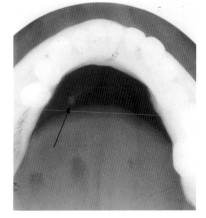

Fig 28-8 Intraoral X-ray view of a stone in the right submandibular duct.

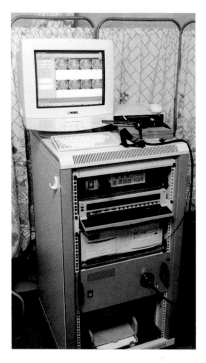

Fig 28-9 Stroboscopic video setup for voice analysis.

Fig 28-10 A fine needle aspirate being taken in outpatients using a special sampling syringe.

CT/Magnetic Resonance Imaging

CT or MRI scanning are particularly helpful in imaging smaller lymph nodes which may be missed on clinical examination.

Fine Needle Aspiration Cytology (FNA)

Fine needle aspiration cytology is very useful if a neck lump is thought to be malignant (see p21) and this can be done in out-patients without anesthetic. There is no evidence of spread of tumor through the skin track caused by the hypodermic needle used for FNA cytology (Fig 28-10). Positive cytology is helpful but negative results cannot be relied on absolutely. The key to good FNA is the expertise of the cytologist.

Ultrasound Scanning

Ultrasound can be very informative in differentiating solid lesions (eg, malignant lymph nodes) from cystic lesions (eg, branchial cysts). This technique is also very helpful in the management of thyroid swellings.

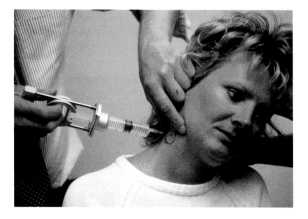

THE SALIVARY GLANDS

Plain X Rays

Plain X rays are of limited value. Fortunately, most submandibular calculi are radio-opaque (Figs 28-8 and 28-11) and can be visualized with appropriate plain X rays.

Sialography

The duct of the parotid or submandibular salivary glands can be cannulated and contrast injected (Figs 28-12 and 28-13). This dis-

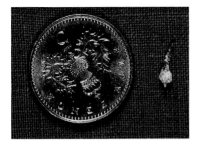

Fig 28-11 The stone that was removed from the patient in Fig 28-8.

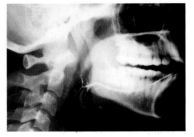

Fig 28-12 A normal submandibular sialogram showing good ductal pattern.

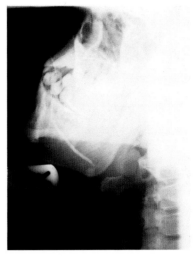

Fig 28-13 Sialogram demonstrating a radio-opaque calculus.

plays the entire ductal system and can be helpful in demonstrating distortion of the ducts by tumor or chronic changes in the gland such as sialectasis.

CT Scanning

CT scanning is of relatively limited value except when an obviously malignant lesion is being assessed for erosion of adjacent bony structures. This technique is, however, very useful when assessing parotid lesions with extension into the parapharyngeal space.

Magnetic Resonance Imaging (MRI)

Magnetic resonance imaging is a superior technique for imaging salivary malignancies—especially those affecting the parotid gland (Fig 28-14). MRI and CT can be combined with sialography.

Fine Needle Aspiration (FNA) Cytology

Fine needle aspiration cytology offers advantages in the assessment of potential tumors as a few cells can be removed in outpatients for microscopic analysis without prejudicing the future management of the patient (unlike open biopsy). Interpretation of salivary cell smears is very difficult, however, and requires an exceptionally high level of expertise. As before, negative results should be interpreted cautiously.

THE THYROID GLAND

Thyroid Function Tests

These are of use in determining whether the patient has a normally functioning gland (euthyroid), a gland functioning below normal (hypothyroid) or an excessively active gland (hyperthyroid). The

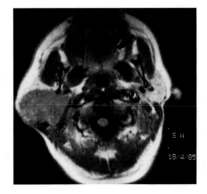

Fig 28-14 A magnetic resonance scan of a large parotid tumor (bones do not show up on MRI scans).

production of thyroxine (T4) and its precursor tri-iodothyronine (T3) are easily measured. In addition it is common practice to measure the level of thyroid-stimulating hormone (TSH).

Autoantibody Tests

The thyroid gland is a common site for autoimmune disease and the levels of thyroid microsomal antibody or anti-thryroglobin antibody can be measured. Because autoimmune disorders are often multiple, a profile of various antibodies is usually measured at once.

Thyroid Ultrasound

This investigation is mandatory in all cases of thyroid nodules and is coupled with *fine needle aspiration cytology* (FNA). If the FNA results are positive, they can be very helpful but caution needs to be exercised in the case of a negative result (false negative rates of up to 5% have been reported).

Thyroid Scans

These are either with radioactive iodine(I^{125}) or technetium(Tc^{99}). These are widely used to ascertain whether a nodule is functioning ("hot") or not functioning ("cold"). Many no longer use this method for planning treatment because a proportion of both types of nodule are malignant.

THE PARATHYROIDS

Biochemistry

Measurements of serum calcium and parathormone (PTH) concentration can be performed. The role of other tests such as scanning are covered in the section on parathyroid diseases.

CHAPTER 29

The Oral Cavity and Pharynx

THE ORAL CAVITY

ACUTE TONSILLITIS

This is usually a bacterial infection caused by a pyogenic group *A. streptococcus.* It is characterized by fever, sore throat, enlargement of the jugulo-digastric lymph node, and dysphagia. White pustules are seen on the palatine tonsils in the area corresponding to the lymphatic follicles—hence the name *follicular tonsillitis.* This acute inflammation is bilateral and almost always sensitive to benzyl or phenoxymethyl penicillin (penicillin V).

Tonsillectomy

This is an effective treatment for recurrent tonsillitis. It is usually considered when attacks have occurred a minimum 4 times each year for at least 18 months. It is also advised for airway obstruction and the sleep apnea syndrome (p169), peritonsillar abscess (p240), and in cases where malignancy is suspected.

Surgical Points

Surgery on the upper part of the airway always carries significant risks—in particular from bleeding and inhalation. Because this operation is often performed in childhood, it is essential to bear in mind that the total blood volume of a child depends on its body weight. An approximate figure is 70-75 ml of blood per kilogram of weight. (This figure is slightly higher in the neonatal period.) From this it follows that a child of 15 kg has a circulating blood volume of just over 1 liter and that a loss of 100 ml certainly requires fluid replacement.

Children, who are bleeding postoperatively, exhibit remarkable maintenance of their blood pressure until fairly late but the pulse rate always rises early on and is one of the most important clinical signs.

> **Key Point:**
> There is no evidence of deleterious long-term immunological side effects from tonsillectomy.

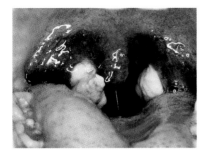

Fig 29-1 The typical appearance of a creamy exudate covering the tonsils in glandular fever. This appearance is virtually diagnostic.

GLANDULAR FEVER

Etiology

This systemic disorder is usually caused by the Epstein-Barr virus but a similar disorder can arise with other infective organisms such as toxoplasma or cytomegalovirus. A small proportion of patients with glandular fever syndrome have a predominantly pharyngeal disease.

Clinical Presentation

The discomfort and dysphagia may be extreme with drooling of saliva and respiratory difficulty (usually inspiratory). The appearance of the throat is typical with a creamy-grey exudate covering both tonsils and appearing confluent (Fig 29-1).

The pharyngeal appearances coupled with a high temperature are virtually diagnostic but the disease can be confirmed by serological testing which should show a positive Paul Bunnel test, an absolute and relative lymphocytosis, and the presence of atypical monocytes in the peripheral blood.

Treatment

Antibiotics are of little value except to prevent secondary bacterial infection—ampicillin should be avoided because of the frequent appearance of a papular rash. Steroids are occasionally required for short-term treatment if the airway is compromised. *If such treatment is necessary it should only be carried out in specialized units because intensive monitoring of the airway is essential.*

Key Point:

Infectious mononucleosis may cause upper airway blockage which can be life-threatening.

Peritonsillar Abscess (Quinsy)

This is fully covered in Emergencies (p240).

HUMAN IMMUNODEFICIENCY VIRUS

Etiology

The human immunodeficiency virus, which is the causative agent of Acquired Immune Deficiency syndrome (AIDS), can affect almost all of the ENT system but it is most likely to be seen in the cervical region or in the oral cavity. This syndrome most often affects intravenous drug users and homosexual males; it is also widespread in certain parts of Africa.

Clinical Presentation

The clinical presentation of HIV infection in the head and neck is very varied but classically, these patients develop multiple oral vesicular ulcers especially due to herpetic infection. Any patient may present with an opportunistic infection such as *Candida* or pneumocystis but Kaposi's sarcoma may also arise in the oral cavity and presents as an elevated or flat erythematous nodule (typically on the palate) with intact overlying mucosa.

Cervical lymphadenopathy is also very frequent and this makes the evaluation of a neck mass in a high risk patient very difficult. The neck nodes are usually enlarged due to follicular hyperplasia but lymphomas and other diseases are seen.

WHITE PATCHES

Any white patch which cannot easily be categorized as anything else is called *Leukoplakia*. This usually refers to a dysplasia of the epithelial cells which is seen in smokers and is premalignant. Other causes of white patches include candida and aphthous ulcers.

> **Key Point:**
> White patches in smokers need urgent specialist attention.

Candida

Infection with *Candida albicans* produces confluent white areas which can be wiped off and are sensitive to antifungals. It is usually seen in patients who have had prolonged antibiotic treatment or who are immunosuppressed. In the developed world candidiasis in the oral cavity and oropharynx is also common in patients using steroid inhalers for asthma. It can usually be cured easily and is prevented by giving advice on inhaler technique.

Aphthous Ulcers

These are small painful ulcers 1–5 mm in size and which may occur in crops throughout the oral cavity but are of unknown origin. They are associated with stress. They may be helped by steroid ointments and may recur over a period of many years.

THE GLOBUS SYNDROME

This is a description (Latin: *globus* = lump) for the feeling of a lump in the throat. It is commoner in women and mostly affects the 30–50 age group. Dysphagia means difficulty in swallowing but these patients rarely have true dysphagia.

Etiology

These patients often have gastroesophageal reflux and spasm of the cricopharyngeus muscle at the pharyngo-oesophageal junction. Other causes may include infected postnasal drip (due to sinusitis), pharyngeal pouch, and carcinoma of the pharynx. Most patients are treated by conservative measures such as antacid

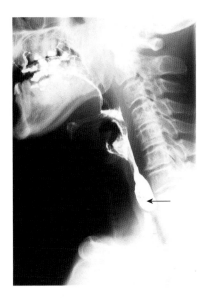

Fig 29-2 A barium study of a pharyngeal pouch (arrowed) visible at the level of C7.

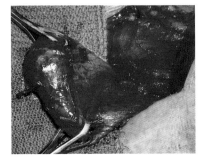

Fig 29-3 Operative view of the pharyngeal pouch seen in Fig 29-2 dissected from the neck and delivered externally prior to excision.

therapy. The original name of globus hystericus is unhelpful and should be abandoned, but psychological studies have shown that sufferers do show abnormal degrees of anxiety and introversion.

Investigation of these patients should include modified barium swallow and videoflouroscopy.

Key Points:

1. The globus syndrome is a difficult diagnosis to make without full investigation.

2. Patients presenting with a lump in the throat need careful evaluation to exclude local disease.

3. Globus is often associated with gastroesophageal reflux.

PHARYNGEAL POUCH

Etiology

This is a false diverticulum arising at the junction of the esophagus and pharynx. A true diverticulum contains all the layers of the organ of origin, but this lesion does not have the muscular layers present. The pharyngeal mucosa herniates posteriorly through a dehiscence between the upper and lower fibres of the inferior constrictor muscle. It typically occurs in males over 60.

Clinical Presentation

A pharyngeal pouch may present with a feeling of a lump in the throat (q.v.) and dysphagia with regurgitation of undigested food into the mouth some hours after eating. Chest infections and coughing are common due to overspill of the contents of the pouch into the airway, especially at night. There may also be some weight loss.

Examination may show some pooling of saliva on indirect or flexible laryngoscopy, but this is usually unremarkable. A barium study usually demonstrates the pouch (Fig 29-2).

Treatment

This may be by an external approach to resect or invaginate the pouch (Fig 29-3), or by endoscopic resection of the partition between pharynx and pouch (most surgeons believe that division of the fibres of cricopharyngeus is essential to prevent recurrence). Recently the endoscopic approach has been improved with the use of stapling guns to divide the partition leading to a much quicker operation with reduced hospital stays (Figs 29-4 and 29-5).

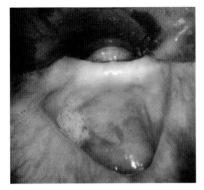

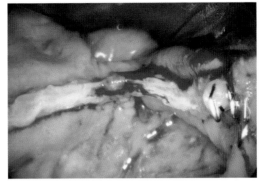

Fig 29-4 Endoscopic view of a pharyngeal pouch. The pouch is below and the smaller opening into the esophagus is above (anterior). The bar dividing the two horizontally is clearly visible.

Fig 29-5 Same patient as shown in Fig 29-4 at the end of the endoscopic stapling procedure. The bar has been divided and some staples are visible.

MALIGNANT TUMORS OF THE PHARYNX (INCLUDING NASOPHARYNX)

Etiology

Tumors in the oral cavity and pharynx are relatively uncommon but it is important to bear in mind that the majority of these tumors can be identified clinically by an ENT specialist. They used to be seen almost exclusively in elderly males but the sex incidence is now changing. This is probably due to the effects of extraneous causative factors such as *cigarette smoking,* which has increased in women in recent years. The consumption of spirits is also almost universal in this group of patients and these toxins damage the entire mucosa of the aerodigestive tract; consequently these tumors do not always arise in isolation. A carcinoma may have extensive surrounding or adjacent mucosal dysplasia and these patients are more likely to develop a second primary malignancy within the aerodigestive tract (including the lungs).

> **Key Points:**
> 1. Almost all cancers in this region are squamous carcinomas.
> 2. Squamous carcinoma of the head and neck usually affects smokers over 40 years.

Nasopharynx

Carcinomas of the nasopharynx are commonly squamous, although they have a tendency to demonstrate a pronounced lymphoid infiltrate. These tumors have a bimodal age distribution, affecting not only older people (over 50) like other head and neck cancers, but also younger patients in the second and third decades. This cancer is also extremely common in the southern Chinese in whom it is the commonest malignant tumor.

Patients present with symptoms of *local disease, cranial nerve involvement at the skull base or with neck metastases.* The *local symptoms* are nasal blockage and bloody discharge with a unilateral middle ear effusion. The *cranial nerves* commonly affected include the oculomotor nerves (III, IV, and VI), and the lower cranial nerves (IX–XII) with trigeminal involvement. One third of these patients present with a lump in the neck—usually *upper deep cervical*.

These tumors can be identified by flexible nasendoscopy, biopsy, and CT or MR scanning and are usually treated by radiotherapy. Epstein Barr surface antigen is a good serological marker of this disease.

Oral Cavity

Oral cavity carcinomas are uncommon except in people who smoke and drink heavily or who chew tobacco or betel nuts (common in Asian communities).

They almost always present as *ulcerative painful lesions* (commonly on the lateral border of the tongue) (Figs 29-6, 29-7, and 29-8) with or without enlargement of regional lymph nodes.

Early tumors are well controlled by radiotherapy or surgery. Advanced carcinomas of the oral cavity and pharynx usually require combined treatment involving radical surgery with resection of tongue, mandible, and adjacent tissue. This type of radical treatment has been made easier in recent years with the advances in reconstructive techniques using skin, muscle, and bone flaps to repair the oral cavity. In this context, the development of microvascular anastamotic techniques in the past 10 years has allowed skin flaps from distant sites such as the groin or forearm to be transplanted into the mouth and neck ("free flaps") (Figs 29-9–29-13). Advanced tumors are usually also treated with radiotherapy in a planned combined fashion with surgery.

Chemotherapy has no proven therapeutic role in the management of squamous carcinoma and its use is mainly confined to clinical trials.

Pharynx

ENT surgeons divide the pharynx into nasopharynx, oropharynx (from the anterior faucial pillar to the tip of the epiglottis), and hypopharynx (from epiglottis to the esophageal inlet at the level of C6) (See Figs 29-14 and 29-15).

Pharyngeal cancers are uncommon except in elderly smokers. They commonly cause *painful dysphagia* and odynophagia (pain in the mouth on swallowing) with or without referred otalgia and can usually be identified on clinical examination, especially with fibreoptic laryngoscopy. They are often advanced at presentation and the overall outlook is poor.

They may be managed by radiotherapy and radical surgery such as pharyngo-laryngo-esophagectomy. This requires replacement of

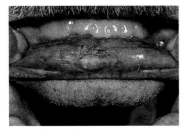

Fig 29-6 A small squamous carcinoma of the lower lip in the midline which was successfully treated by radiotherapy.

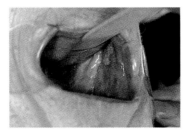

Fig 29-7 A tumor on the right buccal mucosa in a smoker.

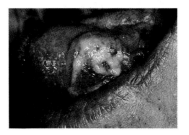

Fig 29-8 A large carcinoma on the lateral border of the tongue treated by radical surgery.

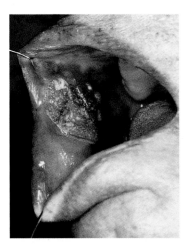

Fig 29-9 A large squamous carcinoma of the right buccal mucosa prior to excision.

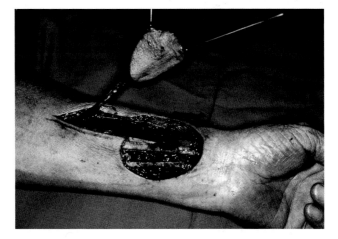

Fig 29-10 A free flap being harvested from the patient's left forearm with attached radial artery and veins. The donor site is closed with a split skin graft.

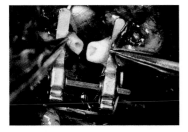

Fig 29-11 A close-up of the radial artery (on the right) about to be anastomosed to the facial artery (on the left).

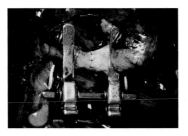

Fig 29-12 A close-up view of the vessels seen in Fig 29-11 after the sutures have been placed.

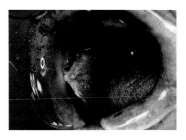

Fig 29-13 Result of treatment in the patient from Fig 29-9 1 week after surgery. Note that the radial forearm skin now replaces the buccal mucosa.

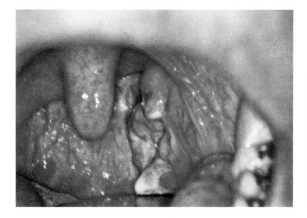

Fig 29-14 Ulcerating carcinoma, left tonsillar region.

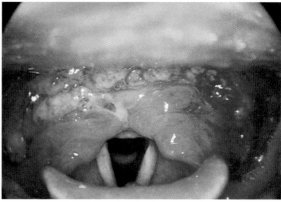

Fig 29-15 Endoscopic view of a postcricoid carcinoma. The ultimate relationship of this tumor to the larynx is clearly seen.

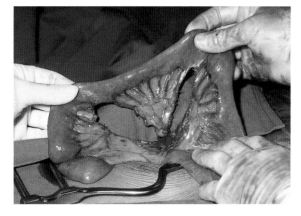

Fig 29-16 Jejunum being mobilized prior to transfer to the neck in a patient with postcricoid carcinoma.

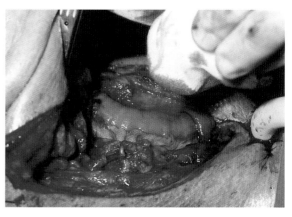

Fig 29-17 Jejunum in situ in the neck. It is sutured to the tongue base above (on the left) and to the stomach below.

the pharynx and esophagus by mobilizing the stomach ("stomach pull-up"), inserting a free jejunal graft, (Figs 9-16 and 29-17), mobilizing the transverse colon, or converting a skin flap into a tube.

Key Point:

Radical operations on terminally ill patients normally fail.

CHAPTER 30

Laryngeal and Voice Disorders

....

THE SYMPTOMS OF LARYNGEAL DISEASE

There are three main symptoms of laryngeal disease: (1) hoarseness, (2) stridor, and (3) aspiration.

1. *Hoarseness.* This is primarily a symptom of laryngeal disease. Occasionally it is a manifestation of distant disease, such as hypothyroidism or lung cancer.

2. *Stridor.* The larynx is the only part of the respiratory tract which contains an entire circle of cartilage—the cricoid cartilage. In addition, the area just below the vocal cords—the subglottis—is the narrowest part of the airway. Obstruction leads to diminished airflow and this leads to turbulence. The turbulent air flowing through a narrowed larynx causes a musical noise called stridor. This is usually *inspiratory stridor* when the blockage is at or above the level of the vocal cords and *biphasic stridor* if the blockage is in the subglottis or in the trachea. *Expiratory stridor* is usually called wheeze and arises because of a similar mechanism obstructing the small airways (eg, in asthma).

3. *Aspiration.* This refers to the inhalation of food or saliva due to failure of the protective function of the larynx. It may manifest as coughing or choking when attempting to swallow and repeated chest infections due to saliva soiling the lungs. It may be seen in patients with an immobile cord due to nerve palsy or tumor and in patients with a pharyngeal pouch.

Aspiration occurs more often with fluids rather than solids, ie, the opposite of dysphagia due to esophageal narrowing. This is because of the greater neuromuscular coordination required to swallow fluids.

Pain: Pain in the larynx is not a specific feature—it may be seen with infection or neoplasia. Referred pain (*to the ear*) is a more worrying feature implying malignancy.

> **Key Point:**
> The larynx is a sphincter through which we breathe and which protects the airway during swallowing. It also acts as the generator of speech.

Signs of Laryngeal Disorder

There are 4 main signs of laryngeal disorder.

1. *Voice abnormalities.* To the experienced specialist abnormalities of voice quality may be quite characteristic—for example, the

Key Point:

Airflow varies inversely with the 4th power of the radius of a tube (Poiseuille's formula), so a small reduction in size of the airway (eg, at the level of the larynx) may have a large effect on airflow.

Key Point:

Laryngitis is not an alternative term for hoarseness.

Table 30-1. Disorders of the Larynx

Specific Voice Disorders
  Mass abnormalities (eg, nodules, polyps)
  Diffuse abnormalities (eg, acute and chronic laryngitis)
  Vocal cord palsy
  Laryngeal cancer
Nonspecific Voice Disorders
  Voice strain
  Functional dysphonia

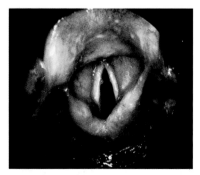

Fig 30-1 Endoscopic view of small vocal nodules (singers' nodules) seen at the junction of the anterior one third and posterior two thirds of the vocal cords.

breathy voice of a vocal cord palsy or the harsh voice of chronic laryngitis. To the lay person, almost any term may be applied to encompass all abnormalities!

Dysphonia: This is merely a description of abnormal voice and not a diagnosis.

Laryngitis: This is a description of a specific appearance of the larynx and cannot be made without viewing it.

2. *Stridor.* The noisy breathing of the stidulous patient is easily detected. This is more common in young children where the airway is smaller (pp235-236). Since the subglottis is the narrowest part of the airway, a small change here may have a disproportionately large effect on airflow.

3. *Mobility.* Occasionally the mobility of the larynx to palpation may be impaired due to tumor, but this is usually a late sign.

4. *Lump in Neck.* Carcinoma of the larynx metastasizes to the neck and this may be one of the presenting signs in advanced cases.

Disorders of the larynx are classified in Table 30-1.

CAUSES OF HOARSENESS

Mass Abnormalities

Vocal Nodules

These are also known as singers' or screamers' nodules (Fig 30-1). They are symmetrical small white swellings on the apposing surface of the true cords, usually situated at the junction of the anterior one third and posterior two thirds. They are the result of poor voice production or chronic overuse—therefore speech therapy is the best treatment. Occasionally they will need to be surgically removed using micro-surgical techniques or endolaryngeal laser surgery followed by speech therapy to correct the underlying errors in voice production.

Papillomata

Respiratory papillomata are rare in adults. They usually occur in children and they tend to spread throughout the tracheabronchial tree airway if not carefully treated. They are of viral origin (human papilloma viruses especially HPV 6 and 11) and are removed by laser surgery, with repetition at regular intervals, coupled with antiviral agents such as interferon. The value of endoscopic laser surgery is that it causes very little scarring and does not appear to facilitate the implantation of the papillomata further down the airway. It is a great advance over earlier, more crude techniques and avoids the need for tracheostomy.

Polyps (Fig 30-2)

Polyps are uncommon and often unilateral. They tend to follow an acute infective episode and will not resolve spontaneously. They require removal by microsurgery or laser treatment.

Diffuse Abnormalities

Acute Laryngitis

This occurs as part of a diffuse upper respiratory infection or as a localized disorder. It is often viral and settles quickly. Active treatment is not essential but steam inhalations are soothing. It does not last more than 3 weeks in the vast majority of cases.

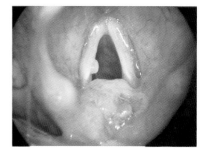

Fig 30-2 A polyp on the posterior part of the left vocal cord.

> **Key Point:**
> Hoarseness lasting more than 3 weeks should always be referred for an ENT opinion in case it is due to an early laryngeal cancer.

Chronic Laryngitis

Chronic laryngitis is divided—like all chronic inflammation—into *chronic specific* and *chronic nonspecific* laryngitis. This separates inflammations due to a known agent such as TB, leprosy, etc. (ie, chronic specific) from those due to an unknown agent.

Chronic specific laryngitis. The identification of laryngitis due to Mycobacteria, Syphilis, fungi, etc is by biopsy. These disorders are now rare in the developed world. Treatment is directed towards the causative organism, eg, dapsone for leprosy.

Chronic nonspecific laryngitis. The main predisposing factors are smoking, chronic upper respiratory sepsis (chronic sinusitis with postnasal drip), and chronic lower respiratory sepsis (chronic obstructive airways disease). In some cases, the laryngeal mucosa may become *dysplastic*—especially over the surface of the true vocal cords. This may be a premalignant condition—hence the need for expert appraisal or laser surgery (eg, using the carbon dioxide laser).

The condition is treated by elimination of any predisposing factors such as smoking and by regular stripping of the affected areas of the vocal cords by microsurgery or by laser surgery using the CO_2 laser.

The risk of malignant change depends on the severity of any dysplasia and continuation of the provoking factors.

> **Key Point:**
> The diagnosis of chronic laryngitis should never be made unless the larynx has been fully assessed by a laryngologist.

Vocal Cord Palsy

This may be unilateral or bilateral. Unilateral is commonest and left cord palsy is the most frequently encountered.

Unilateral. Unilateral left vocal cord palsy is the commonest because the left recurrent laryngeal nerve pursues a long intrathoracic course arching round the aorta, and is commonly involved in neoplasms involving the left hilum. Since lung cancer is the commonest single cancer, it must be considered first. Other lesions can cause a similar effect including cancer of the thyroid, esophagus, and nasopharynx. Neurological lesions should also come into the differential diagnosis (see Table 30-2).

Bilateral. Bilateral cord palsies are uncommon and tend to occur after thyroid surgery or head injuries.

Key Points:

1. Left cord palsy is usually considered due to a carcinoma of the lung until proven otherwise.

2. Although cancer of the lung is the commonest single cause of left cord palsy, it is not the commonest cause of hoarseness.

Treatment. The larynx often compensates in cases of unilateral palsy. If no improvement in voice quality occurs after 3 to 6 months, improvements can be achieved by laryngeal surgery techniques which are known collectively as *phonosurgery*.

Unilateral palsies. These may be managed by injecting Teflon paste or bovine collagen into the affected side to bring it closer to the midline. This may be injected *transcutaneously* directly into the vocal fold under local anaesthesia with fiberoptic nasoendoscopic

---

Table 30-2. Causes of Vocal Cord Palsy

Cause	Cord	Comments
Iatrogenic	Following thyroidectomy/ neck surgery/chest surgery	Common
Bronchial cancer	Left vocal cord	Common
Skull base lesions	Either cord	
Thyroid/esophageal cancer	Either cord	Clinical examination
Cardiomegaly	Left vocal cord	Esp. left atrium
Neurological diseases	Either cord	Multiple sclerosis
Idiopathic	Usually left	Common
		Often follows viral infections

control. Alternatively this can be done directly into the vocal fold under general anaesthesia using a rigid endoscope. Since the intracordal injections are not easily reversed, new techniques have been developed to mobilize a part of the laryngeal framework and its associated soft tissues and bring them surgically nearer the midline. This is known as *thyroplasty* or *laryngeal framework surgery*. In type I thyroplasty for unilateral palsies, the thyroid cartilage is exposed and precisely fenestrated. A preformed implant (made from a variety of materials such as cartilage or silastic) is then inserted to push the vocal fold medially. This technique can be done under local aneasthesia which allows precise positioning of the implant by visualising the larynx preoperatively and asking the patient to phonate. Thyroplasty is not only reversible by removing the implant but also preserves the mucosa across the vocal fold which produces a much better voice quality.

Bilateral palsies. In *bilateral palsies* the cords are often close to the midline (paramedian position), and therefore the airway is already compromised. These patients, therefore, often require tracheostomy. Laryngeal surgery may be carried out on one arytenoid cartilage—either to move it to a more lateral position or to excise it altogether with the CO_2 laser as an endoscopic procedure. Some surgeons advocate reinnervation procedures for the paralyzed larynx—eg, rotating in a nerve-muscle combination from the neck. Any strap muscle can be used but the omohyoid appears to be the most useful. However, these techniques have not yet found widespread acceptance.

Key Point:
In bilateral cord palsy there is always a "trade-off" between improving the airway and restoring voice quality.

Key Point:
Idiopathic cord palsy can only be diagnosed after all other causes have been excluded.

Laryngeal Cancer

Carcinomas of the larynx are predominantly squamous carcinomas and this is one of the commonest head and neck cancers, almost always occurring in elderly smokers. Over the past 20 years the sex incidence has changed and 20% of these tumors now occur in women. As in the oral cavity and pharynx, the normal stratified squamous epithelium of the larynx can exhibit a range of changes from mild dysplasia to carcinoma in situ to invasive carcinoma. (Fig 30-3). The majority of laryngeal carcinomas (55%)

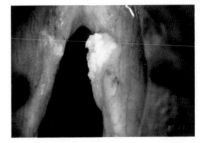

Fig 30-3 Endoscopic view of the larynx with marked dysplasia and keratosis on the anterior part of the right vocal cord.

arise from the vocal cords—ie, glottic. About 40% arise from the supraglottis and a small proportion are primarily subglottic.

Presentation

Because of the sites of origin, patients almost always present with *hoarseness* and this is of great importance because early cancers have a 90% 5-year cure rate. The cure rate drops dramatically with increased size of tumor at presentation.

Staging

Laryngeal cancers are staged according to the classic TNM system. The importance of this is that the prognosis changes with different stages and that it allows comparison of treatment results from different techniques and different centres.

T1   Tumor confined to the vocal cords with *normal* mobility.

T2   Tumor in two sites, eg, glottis and supraglottis, with normal or *impaired* mobility of cords.

T3   Tumor confined to the larynx with a *fixed* vocal cord.

T4   Tumor outside the larynx (eg, pyriform fossa).

Treatment

Early tumors (T1&T2). The vast majority are treated primarily by radiotherapy for cure, with surgery usually reserved for recurrence. It is now being appreciated that surgery is equally effective for small tumors and can be done endoscopically (eg, with laser-assisted techniques). Surgery has the great advantage that it is completed much more quickly than a typical course of radiotherapy, which can last for several weeks (Fig 30-4).

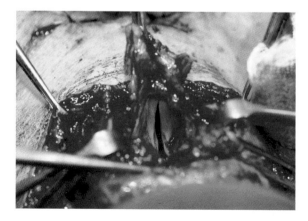

Fig 30-4 A supraglottic laryngectomy. The vocal cords are clearly visible as the excision nears completion.

Late tumors (T3 & T4). Large tumors tend not to respond so well to radiotherapy. Accordingly, most centers advocate radical surgery with adjuvant radiotherapy postoperatively. Laryngeal carcinomas tend to spread via lymphatics to the cervical nodes (p219) and their involvement is a poor prognostic sign. Accordingly all cases with established neck metastases (N+) are automatically in this category even if the primary tumor is small.

Chemotherapy is not particularly helpful and tends only to be used in otherwise untreatable cases or in controlled trials.

Key Point:

T1 and T2 laryngeal cancers have an 85–90% 5-year survival rate.

Laryngectomy

This radical operation for advanced or recurrent cancer involves a permanent interruption of the connection between the upper aerodigestive tract (nose, mouth) and lower respiratory tract (lungs). Part or all of the thyroid gland is usually removed at the same time (Fig 30-5) and the patient breathes through a tracheal stump, which is sutured to the neck skin (Fig 30-6). After laryngectomy, the patient cannot immerse his neck in water—even to have a bath or shower. Well motivated patients, however, can overcome even this problem (Fig 30-7).

Key Point:

Remember to check T4/Calcium status regularly in patients who have undergone laryngectomy.

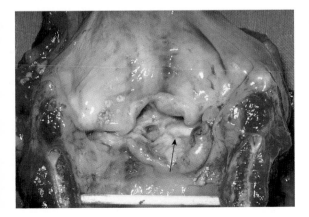

Fig 30-5 A typical laryngectomy specimen photographed close up and demonstrating a large ulcerative tumor at the level of the true cord (arrowed). The specimen has been split in the midline posteriorly and is being propped open by a small wooden stick at the lower margin of the picture.

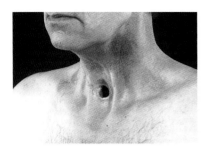

Fig 30-6 A tracheal stoma following total laryngectomy. The patient's lungs have no other connection to the outside world.

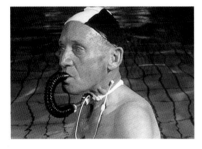

Fig 30-7 A rather complex device being worn by a laryngectomy sufferer to enable him to go swimming. Note that the patient has managed to reconnect his nasal and oral airway with his trachea.

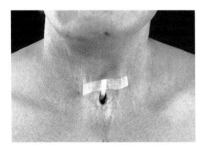

Fig 30-8 A similar patient to Fig 30-7 but with a small Blom-Singer valve in the stoma being held in place by a piece of white tape.

Thyroxine and calcium supplements need to be taken orally for life if the whole thyroid gland has been removed.

Vocal Rehabilitation

The loss of the larynx (vocal generator) does not prevent speech production as long as an alternative source of vibrating air can be found in the pharynx. Three alternatives are available: (1) artificial devices which cause vibration of air in the oral cavity or pharynx—usually battery-powered; (2) voice production may be restored in some patients by regurgitating air into the pharynx and then using this as a source for articulation (*esophageal speech*); (3) a small channel can be created in the tracheal stoma to allow exhaled air to pass into the pharynx via a one-way valve (tracheoesophageal speech). This involves the implantation of a small device such as a Blom-Singer valve (Fig 30-8). These latter techniques have now become widespread.

NONSPECIFIC VOICE DISORDERS

Voice Strain

This is quite common in people who use their voices a lot. It is associated with incomplete closure of the vocal cords at some point along their length. A version of this also occurs in some patients who are on treatment with inhaled steroids when the cords present a "bowed" appearance on attempted phonation.

Treatment is by voice rest and speech therapy.

Functional Dysphonia

Functional dysphonia usually covers all conditions where there is no obvious disorder and the larynx appears to be moving normally. There may be a number of problems underlying the dysphonia which are not immediately apparent ranging, from excess muscle tension in the strap muscles of the neck to stress, emotional conflict, personality disorder, or frank psychiatric illness. It is commonly seen in young women. Speech therapy is the most useful treatment, although a psychologist may be required in some cases.

CHAPTER 31

Neck Diseases

LUMPS IN THE NECK: GENERAL COMMENTS

The correct diagnosis of a lump in the neck requires a careful history and examination. Most clinicians will gain 90% of their diagnostic information from this alone.

Site, size, duration, and consistency of the mass are essential items of information. Midline swellings are usually congenital dermoids (Figs 31-1 and 31-2) or of thyroid origin. Masses along the line of the sternomastoid muscle are usually either lymph nodes or branchial cysts (see Table 31-1). Fluctuant painful swellings are usually due to infected abscesses. Remember the surgical sieve: ie, congenital or acquired. If acquired, is it infectious, inflammatory, endocrine, or neoplastic?

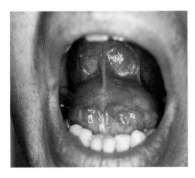

Fig 31-1 A large midline dermoid visible in the floor of the mouth.

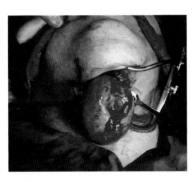

Fig 31-2 The dermoid from Fig 31-1 being delivered externally after an incision below the chin.

Table 31-1. Causes of Lumps in the Neck

Midline	Lateral
Thyroid anomalies	Lymphangiomas (cystic hygroma)
Dermoid cysts	Lymph nodes
	Branchial cysts
	Neurogenic
	Carotid body tumor

LYMPH NODES

Small rubbery lymph nodes are typical of local infection, especially in children, but large nodes (more than 3 cm) or multiple nodes are highly suggestive of malignancy (Fig 31-3).

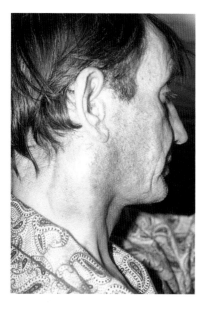

Fig 31-3 A large right upper neck lump (upper deep cervical) in a patient with a carcinoma of the tonsil (see also Fig 29-14).

LYMPHOMA

A lymphoma is common in young adults but squamous carcinoma is common in older patients (over 50 years). In view of this, excision biopsy is not appropriate until a full ENT examination has been performed to identify the primary tumor (see Table 31-2). Ideally this should be done under general anesthetic. If no tumor is evident, biopsy of the nasopharynx, posterior third of tongue, and tonsillectomy should be performed as this may reveal a submucosal primary carcinoma. Treatment of squamous carcinoma of the neck is usually by a radical neck dissection rather than radiotherapy.

Key Point:

A lump in the neck in an adult is due to a tumor arising in the pharynx or larynx until proven otherwise.

Table 31-2. Disadvantages of Biopsy of Neck Lumps without ENT Assessment

1. The patient may feel the lump has been removed and not attend for further follow-up.
2. The neck has a scar, which complicates future clinical assessment.
3. Tumor seeding may have occurred into the neck tissues and the skin.
4. The pathology report of "metastatic squamous carcinoma of unknown origin" is of no value to the patient or clinician and represents a wasted general anesthetic.

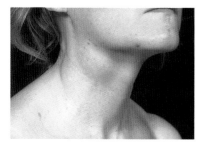

Fig 31-4 A branchial cyst in the right upper neck.

BRANCHIAL CYST

This is a malformation which usually presents in the upper neck in early or middle adulthood. A swelling is detected at the junction of the upper third and the middle third of the sternomastoid muscle on its anterior border (Fig 31-4). On initial presentation there may be an acute illness due to infection of the cyst and the diagnosis can be confirmed by ultrasound and aspiration of contents. Treatment is by excision. An acutely inflamed cyst should never be incised as this will convert it into a branchial sinus, which is much more difficult to excise adequately.

LYMPHOMA

The mass of lymphatic tissue around the oropharynx known as Waldeyer's ring (ie, in the area of the tonsil) may be affected in

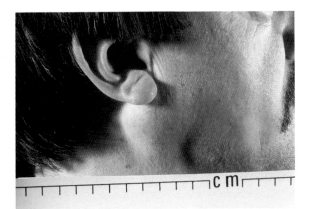

Fig 32-5 A swelling over the angle of the right mandible in a patient with a pleomorphic adenoma of the parotid gland.

SIALORRHOEA

Some patients—especially mentally handicapped children—suffer from drooling of saliva. A full ENT assessment is required and surgery such as adenoidectomy may help. In some cases, the submandibular ducts need to be transposed posteriorly to lie near the tonsil; this may be coupled with ligation of one of the parotid ducts.

BENIGN SALIVARY TUMORS

Pleomorphic Adenoma

This is the most common tumor of salivary tissue and the most frequent tumor in the parotid gland; it is also known as a mixed parotid tumor. Pathologically it consists of epithelial and myoepithelial cells (hence the old name of "mixed tumor"). Pleomorphic adenomata account for 70% of parotid masses and approximately 40% of submandibular swellings. They are slightly more common in women and the maximum incidence is at 40-50 years. Malignant degeneration is rare and tends to be seen in patients with a long history.

Clinical Presentation

These lesions usually present as a lump which for years has been slowly enlarging, situated over or just behind the angle of the mandible (Figs 32-5 and 32-6). Pain or other symptoms are rare. The swelling is firm, nontender, and not fixed to overlying structures/mucosa. No facial nerve signs are found.

Treatment

Treatment is impossible without histological assessment. Accordingly, the correct treatment is excision biopsy of all these lumps

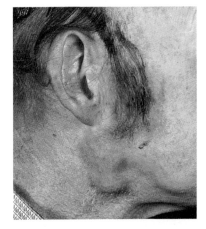

Fig 32-6 Large benign parotid tumor.

(basic surgical principle). In the parotid region, this usually involves superficial parotidectomy with facial nerve preservation. Recurrences are nodular, multi-centric, and usually fixed and are said to be much less likely if formal superficial parotidectomy is performed at the time of the original operation.

Excision of recurrences involves greater risk of surgical damage to the facial nerve than primary surgery.

Postoperative radiotherapy (RT). Radiotherapy may be valuable if a minor salivary gland tumor has been incompletely removed or if tumor seeding has occurred intraoperatively. The principle of using radiotherapy for benign disease is contentious as the long-term effects of RT also include degeneration of normal tissue into malignancy (eg, RT-induced sarcomas).

Suprafacial parotidectomy versus lumpectomy. Some surgeons have advocated simple excision of the parotid lump ("lumpectomy"). The basic surgical principles, which should always be observed, are demonstration of the facial nerve and removal of the tumor mass with a cuff of "normal" tissue. This is best accomplished by suprafacial parotidectomy (Fig 32-7).

Warthin's Tumor

Clinical Presentation

This is also known as an adenolymphoma. It is more common in men over the age of 60 (male:female = 5:1) and is occasionally bilateral (less than 10%). Warthin's tumors represent one tenth of parotid swellings and this is the most commonly affected gland—the lower pole of the gland is usually affected and has a typical cystic feel and ovoid shape. Symptoms are rare and these tumors usually present as slowly growing asymptomatic lumps.

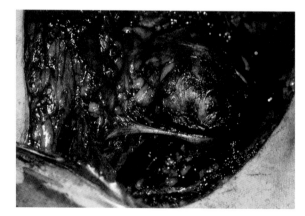

Fig 32-7 A left parotid dissection that clearly demonstrates branches of the facial nerve lying immediately superficial to the neoplasm. This demonstrates why all parotid lumps should be approached via a formal facial nerve dissection.

Treatment

Treatment is as for any parotid swelling. These tumors are encapsulated and have an excellent prognosis.

Hemangioma

These usually occur in children under 1 year. They are commonest in the parotid gland and most regress spontaneously, so are not treated unless actually enlarging. If excised, they rarely recur.

Lymphangioma

These are similar to haemangiomas and they usually occur under the age of 2 years and in the parotid. They should be treated conservatively.

MALIGNANT TUMORS

Adenoid Cystic Carcinoma

This is the most common malignancy of salivary tissue and has a very characteristic clinical pattern. It has a predeliction for neural tissue, and hence, nerve palsy and pain are common early symptoms.

Clinical Presentation

The age of onset is 20-60 years, and they are more common in women. Adenoid cystic carcinoma represents the commonest malignancy in the submandibular or minor salivary glands and 30% of all salivary malignancies. The predilection for neural spread causes early neuropathy and pain which is out of proportion to the size of the lesion. They tend to recur after many years (5-15 years) partly because of their tendency to grow proximally up nerves. They also have a tendency for blood-borne spread to the lungs (cannon ball metastases).

Treatment

These tumors are not radio-sensitive and are usually treated by primary radical surgery. The natural history is of a slowly but inevitably recurring malignancy. Aggressive treatment is justified but ultimate cure is very unlikely.

> **Key Points: Adenoid Cystic Carcinoma**
> 1. It is more common in women.
> 2. Facial nerve involvement and pain are common.
> 3. Late metastases are common.

Mucoepidermoid Tumor

These make up 5-10% of salivary tumors and 90% of them arise in the parotid. They may occur at any age, including childhood. Mucoepidermoid tumors are slow growing with a tendency to local recurrence, but regional lymph-node spread is seen in up to 30% of cases and distant spread in 15%. There is a distinct histological variation: low grade tumors have a 90% 5-year survival rate and high grade tumors 30% 5-year survival rate.

Treatment is usually managed by local excision but radiotherapy is used as an adjunct for high grade lesions.

Adenocarcinoma

These form 3% of parotid tumors and 10% of extraparotid salivary tumors. They usually arise after the age of 30 and occur equally in both sexes. They are also occasionally seen in children.

Treatment

These tumors are best treated by *radical local excision* as they are not radio-sensitive, but distant metastases occur.

Squamous Carcinoma

These are rare in salivary tissue and are twice as common in men as women. They usually occur in elderly patients (over 60 years) and grow rapidly, involving nerves, skin (Fig 32-8), and regional lymph nodes. The prognosis is poor.

Treatment

Treatment consists of radical excision and radiotherapy.

Lymphoma

Three-quarters of salivary lymphomas are found in the parotid gland. There is usually a short history (less than 6 months). Pain and facial palsy are uncommon. As with all lymphomas, clinical stage and histological subtype determine survival. Median survival is 4 years.

Metastatic Carcinoma

Occasionally a malignant parotid mass may be a secondary deposit. The commonest primary site is the scalp but other areas to be considered include breast and kidney.

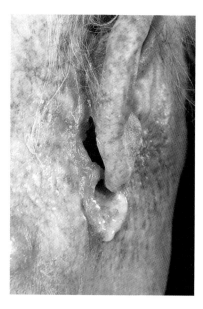

Fig 32-8 Squamous carcinoma of the parotid causing skin breakdown and fistulization following unsuccessful primary radiotherapy.

Key Point:

In children mucoepidemoid carcinomas and pleomorphic adenomas are the commonest tumors but vascular lesions predominate in infancy.

Key Point:

Tumors of the minor salivary glands have a higher tendency to be malignant.

CHAPTER 33

Thyroid Gland Disorders

··

GOITER

This really just means enlargement of the gland and does not predict the disease. However, it has commonly been associated with the enlargement found in geographical areas where iodine is in short supply and hence with hypothyroidism.

HYPOTHYROIDISM

This may be *primary* hypothyroidism due to abnormal uptake of iodine, synthesis of abnormal thyroxine, or absence of the gland (eg, after surgical resection with laryngectomy p232).

    Secondary hypothyroidism occurs when the pituitary fails to produce TSH to stimulate the thyroid gland. The symptoms include cold intolerance, drowsiness, and a hoarse voice.

HYPERTHYROIDISM

This may be due to primary hyperthyroidism or due to a toxic adenoma. The symptoms include irritability, insomnia, sweating, palpitations, and so on. Such patients usually have a tachycardia and may develop eye signs, such as lid lag and exophthalmos, which may require surgical decompression (p118). The mainstay of treatment is with antithyroid drugs such as carbimazole.

THYROGLOSSAL TRACT CYSTS

Embryology

The thyroid gland descends early in fetal life from the base of the tongue towards its eventual position in the lower neck. At the time of descent, the hyoid has not been formed and the track of descent may pass in front of, through, or behind the eventual position of the body of the hyoid. Thyroglossal tract cysts represent persistence of this track and may be found anywhere in the midline from the tongue base to the lower neck. Caution needs to be exercised as

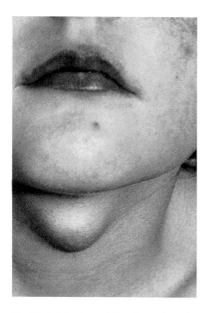

Fig 33-1 A typical midline thyroglossal cyst.

these abnormalities are sometimes the only functioning thyroid tissue in the body.

Presentation

Cysts almost always arise in the midline (Fig 33-1) and may also present at a time of acute infection. The classical description is of a cyst which moves upwards on swallowing and tongue protrusion, but this merely confirms attachment to the hyoid bone.

Treatment

Excision is the best treatment, but the body of the hyoid bone and the suprahyoid track must be excised in order to prevent recurrence (Sistrunk operation). These abnormalities may also present as sinuses following infection.

SOLITARY THYROID NODULE

Clinical Presentation

Most patients will have no features of biochemical thyroid disease, but care should also be taken to elicit any history of neck irradiation in childhood as the thyroid gland is known to be very susceptible to malignant change even 20-30 years later. In addition, a family history of thyroid cancer raises the possibility of medullary carcinoma (see below) and multiple endocrine neoplasia syndrome (MEN), which is an inherited condition.

Management

The critical question for any solitary thyroid lump is whether or not it is really part of a multinodular goitre (always benign) with the other nodules remaining clinically impalpable. This question is answered by *ultrasound* examination. This has the added advantage of demonstrating if a genuinely solitary nodule is cystic or solid. Cystic nodules can then be aspirated for cytology. Solid nodules can be aspirated or excised.

Radioisotope scanning with technetium 99m (Tc 99m) can be used instead of ultrasound to determine whether a nodule is hot or cold (ie takes up radioisotope or not). Hot nodules are said to be benign and cold nodules to have a risk of malignancy of 8%-20%. However, where fine needle aspiration is practiced, isotope scanning can be reserved for patients who are toxic (hyperthyroid) or those in whom metastases are being sought for treatment with radioiodine.

Surgery is useful in

1. all cases of solid or cystic nodules with equivocal cytology; and

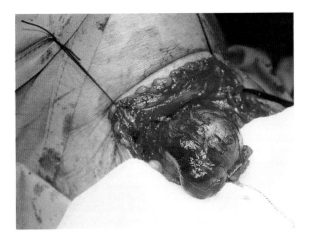

Fig 33-2 Large thyroid mass being delivered peroperatively.

2. other cases where patient preference, symptoms of pressure, or other clinical features dictate.

   Observation is useful in large nodules which are part of a mutinodular goiter where the patient is euthyroid and has no symptoms of pressure (Fig 33-2).

MALIGNANT THYROID DISEASE

Papillary Carcinoma

Clinical Presentation

This is the commonest tumor of the thyroid gland and may represent up to 60% of thyroid cancers. It is usually seen in young adults and typically spreads to cervical lymph nodes (40%). This disease in the lymph nodes was, at one time, known as "lateral aberrant thyroid" because of the apparently well-differentiated nature of the tumors. Other metastases are found rarely—pulmonary in less than 5% of patients.

These tumors may be under TSH control. *Histologically* some follicular elements are usually found, but all tumors with any papillary features are treated as papillary even if they are mainly follicular.

Treatment

If a single small nodule is found, it is usually treated by lobectomy. A total thyroidectomy is not the treatment of choice for this condition with or without lymph nodes.

Follicular Carcinoma

Clinical Presentation

These represent 25% of thyroid carcinomas and occur in older people (20-50 years). They typically spread by blood-borne emboli, especially to bone and lung (cannonball metastases). *Histologically,* the tumors mimic typical glandular acini. Nodal spread is rare (less than 5%).

Treatment

The treatment is always total thyroidectomy. Radioactive iodine is not given routinely, but only in the event that secondaries actually appear.

Key Points:

1. The more follicular a tumor the better its differentiation, and therefore the more likely it is to take up radioiodine.

2. Any swelling over 5 cm should be managed by total thyroidectomy.

Medullary Carcinoma

Clinical Presentation

This is an uncommon tumor of neural crest origin and arises from the parafollicular or C cells. These cells are part of a "family" of cells throughout the body known as Amine Precursor Uptake and Decarboxylase cells (APUD). In the thyroid they are responsible for calcitonin secretion and levels of this hormone may be elevated. Twenty-five percent of medullary carcinomas are familial and 75% are sporadic. Most familial cases have an oncogene mutation and all members of a family should be screened. This can be done by giving the patient either alcohol or gastrin. Serum calcitonin is measured and if it rises, the condition is confirmed. Spread to regional nodes is common. There may be multiple endocrine neoplasia (MEN) with this, eg, phaeochromocytoma. Medullary carcinomas are usually slow growing and may be associated with MEN IIa and IIb: phaeochromocytomas and/or parathyroid tumors.

Treatment

The entire gland should be excised because the C cells are scattered and the disease is often multicentric. Radiotherapy and chemotherapy may also be used.

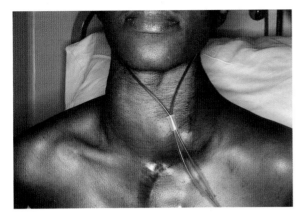

Fig 33-3 A huge neck swelling caused by an anaplastic carcinoma of the thyroid in a young woman with gross tracheal and laryngeal deviation clearly seen.

Anaplastic Carcinoma

This usually occurs in patients over the age of 60 and is usually fatal within 2 years. The tumor typically undergoes rapid enlargement with symptoms of stridor or dyspnoea and often causes regional lymph node enlargement, although these can be obscured by massive primary disease (Fig 33-3).

Treatment is mainly palliative, although radical surgery and RT occasionally produce a good result.

THE PARATHYROIDS

The 4 parathyroid glands usually lie in relation to the posterior surface of the thyroid gland. They are involved in calcium homeostasis and are not uncommonly the site of benign adenoma formation.

Hyperparathyroidism

Primary hyperparathyroidism is due to an excess of parathormone secretion which results in hypercalcaemia. In approx 80% of cases it is caused by a solitary adenoma in one parathyroid gland. About 15% of patients have diffuse hyperplasia of all the parathyroid tissue (this may be hereditary and can be seen with multiple endocrine neoplasia). Less than 5% have multiple adenomas and less than 1% have parathyroid carcinoma.

Presentation

The clinical symptoms of hypercalcaemia are variable and include musculoskeletal (tiredness, bone pain, arthralgia), genitourinary (polyuria, stone formation), gastrointestinal (dry mouth, thirst, anorexia, vomiting), and neurologic (drowsiness/stupor, confusion, blurred vision).

Key Point:
The recurrent laryngeal and superior laryngeal nerves are at especial risk during thyroidectomy.

Investigation

The diagnosis is made by biochemical tests, especially measurement of parathormone (PTH) concentration. Tests to localize the abnormal nodule prior to surgery exist but are not mandatory except in cases where neck exploration has already been negative. Ultrasound can be helpful as can a technetium thallium subtraction scan.

Treatment

The treatment is by exploratory neck surgery and removal of the adenoma. The recurrent laryngeal nerve is at risk as in thyroid surgery. Postoperative hypocalcaemia is common but is usually transient.

CHAPTER 34

Emergencies

STRIDOR

Stridor means noisy breathing. It may be inspiratory or expiratory or biphasic. Inspiratory stridor is usually due to an obstruction at or above the vocal cords. Expiratory stridor is usually from the lower respiratory tract (eg, wheeze). Two-way stridor is usually due to severe obstruction or disease of large airways such as the trachea or main bronchi.

Stridor in Children

Newborn infants or children in the first year of life presenting with stridor should always be assessed clinically, with a full history and examination if the infant's condition will permit. The most common cause of stridor in this age group is *laryngomalacia* (also called congenital laryngeal stridor), but this is not the only cause of this symptom. A multidisciplinary team of anesthesiologist, pediatrician, and otolaryngologist is required to manage these children.

Assessment of an Infant With Stridor

N.B. If a child is cyanosed, it may be impossible to go through the following routine.

History. The phase of stridor and its relationship to activities such as crying, swallowing, etc, are important. Does the child only become distressed and blue when active or when in certain positions? (suggests laryngomalacia). Is the cry weak or otherwise abnormal? (suggests vocal fold palsy). Is the problem exacerbated by feeding? (suggests vascular ring or tracheoesophageal-fistula in the neonate). Is the problem only apparent in conjunction with an upper respiratory infection and is the stridor biphasic? (suggests congenital subglottic stenosis).

Examination. Look at the child at rest before moving or handling it. Once a baby starts to cry, it may be impossible to study its resting pattern for some time! Then ask the mother to move the baby

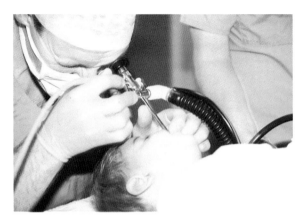

Fig 34-1 An infant undergoing rigid bronchoscopy to determine the cause of stridor. The surgeon is using an endoscope with a Hopkins rod light source.

into different positions, such as face down and supine, and again study its respiratory pattern and level of distress. A transcutaneous oximeter, if available, is helpful here. Then examine the whole child looking for any evidence of external congenital abnormalities before examining the throat. Look inside the mouth and check the palate, tongue, and lower jaw. Always try to watch the child being fed and auscultate the trachea and chest.

Investigations. Oximetry is invaluable. A plain lateral neck X ray and a P-A chest film should always be obtained if the child's condition permits. This may be the best pointer to confirm a foreign body (q.v.). A contrast swallow will identify any vascular abnormalities compressing the trachea (eg, double aortic arch). *Examination under anaesthetic* (Fig 34-1) is an essential tool for any child whose diagnosis remains in doubt, but this requires the utmost skill and close cooperation between surgeon and anesthetist. *Any infant being subjected to rigid laryngoscopy and bronchoscopy may have to have an immediate tracheostomy to establish or maintain an airway.*

Acute Infective Stridor

In the young child this may be due to croup (laryngotracheobronchitis) or acute epiglottitis. These are potentially life-threatening and may need to be managed intensively in hospital. Occasionally the symptoms may be difficult to separate from an inhaled foreign body (see Table 34-1).

Table 34-1. Differential Diagnosis of Acute Pediatric Stridor

	Croup	Epiglottitis	Foreign Body
Age	Under 2 yrs	Over 2 yrs	Any age
History	Slow	Rapid	Rapid
Temperature	Elevated	Elevated	Normal
Cough	Typical bark	None	Spasms

Croup (Laryngotracheobronchitis). This is usually of slower onset, with evidence of general systemic upset. It occurs mostly in young children (under 2 years). The child will usually have inspiratory stridor and hoarseness with a typical barking cough. It is viral in origin and cases may therefore occur in clusters.

Acute Epiglottitis. Usually of much quicker onset and tends to occur in slightly older children, ie, 2 years and over. Rapid progression of stridor with drooling of saliva often occurs. This condition is due to infection with *Haemophilus influenzae*. It is occasionally seen in adults. Where vaccination is practiced, the incidence of acute epiglottitis has declined dramatically.

Both of these disorders may require intensive management with humidification, continuous oximetry to monitor oxygen saturation, and sometimes emergency intubation or tracheostomy. *Restlessness and tachycardia may be signs of hypoxia.*

A lateral neck X ray may be helpful in demonstrating a swollen epiglottis but a very sick child may require immediate management. Tracheostomy may be required if intubation fails but this is also fraught with danger.

Key Point:
Children with epiglottitis may develop airway obstruction rapidly. Insertion of a spatula into the mouth may precipitate acute airway obstruction in a child with epiglottitis and is best avoided.

Key Point:
If in doubt about a child who has stridor, it should be assessed by experienced staff in a hospital.

Foreign Bodies

Foreign bodies may be inhaled and may be very difficult to identify clinically in small children. Children under the age of four are particularly eager to put things into their mouths, which can then be accidentally inhaled. It is commoner for foreign bodies to go down the right main bronchus than the left because it is anatomically slightly more vertical. Plain X rays of the chest are mandatory (Fig 34-2).

Diagnosis. The history is the most important component of the diagnosis but may be impossible to elicit. Particular features are recurrent cough of recent origin (with or without wheezing) or unexplained bronchitis, fever, or toxaemia. Small children are particularly tempted by brightly coloured bits of plastic (eg, from

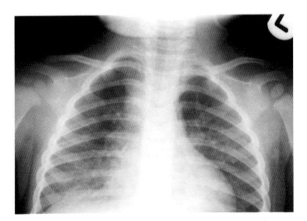

Fig 34-2 Patchy shadowing in right lung field following inhalation of a peanut.

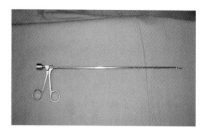

Fig 34-3 Specialized optical forceps for removal of endobronchial foreign bodies.

toys) and by vegetable matter such as peanuts. Where possible, an idential foreign body should be studied. Plain X rays of the chest are mandatory but special tests such as CT scans are not usually required. Bronchoscopy may be required to exclude this as a cause of mediastinal shift or localized pulmonary collapse (Fig 34-3).

Stridor in Adults

Stridor in adults rarely progresses as rapidly as in children. Although they may suffer from infection, the main worry is laryngeal cancer. The diagnosis can usually be made by indirect or fiberoptic laryngoscopy but expert assessment is required.

TRACHEOSTOMY

This is a procedure to *relieve airway obstruction* or to *protect the airway* by fashioning a direct entrance to the trachea through the skin of the neck (see Table 34-2). The tracheostomy may be temporary or permanent and is nowadays usually done following endotracheal intubation. Emergency tracheostomy—when the patient is *in extremis* and the larynx cannot be intubated—is a very difficult procedure and should not be embarked upon lightly. Alternatives exist such as inserting a large intravenous cannula into the cricothyroid membrane, which lies in the midline just below the Adam's apple (*cricothyroidotomy* or *mini-tracheostomy*).

The standard operation involves a transverse neck incision, separation of the strap muscles, and displacement or transfixion of the thyroid isthmus which overlies the trachea. The trachea is incised (Fig 34-4) and initially cannulated with a cuffed plastic tube (Fig 34-5), which may be changed for an uncuffed plastic or silver tube 2-3 days later.

Table 34-2. Tracheostomy

Indications	Example
Relief of upper airway obstruction—Actual	Inhaled foreign body Large Laryngeal tumor Acute infection in a child
Relief of upper airway obstruction—Potential	After major mouth or pharyngeal surgery
Protection of lower airway—Actual	Overspill of saliva in head-injured patients
Protection of lower airway—Potential	Patients requiring artificial ventilation due to respiratory paralysis, eg, drugs, Guillain-Barré syndrome

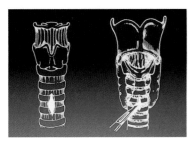

Fig 34-4 A diagram illustrating the site of a tracheal incision for a tracheostomy. Note that the cricoid cartilage and first tracheal ring are inviolate.

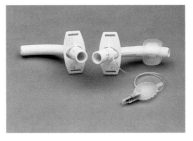

Fig 34-5 Silastic tracheostomy tubes. The one on the left is without a cuff. The tube on the right shows a cuff inflated and is suitable for patients undergoing artificial ventilation—eg, in intensive care.

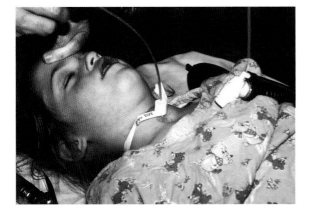

Fig 34-6 An infant undergoing suction of secretions, which were causing airway problems.

Care of Tracheostomies

Highly skilled nursing is required to ensure the lumen of the tracheostomy tube does not become obstructed. Regular humidification and suction (Fig 34-6) are essential. If a patient becomes distressed, always check that pulmonary secretions are not crusted in the lumen by inserting a suction catheter. If this fails, then change the tube (Fig 34-7). Patients who require artificial ventilation or protection of the airway from overspill of saliva need a cuffed tube and cannot change to an uncuffed plastic or silver tube. The latter have the advantage that it may be possible for the patient to speak normally if the tube has the appropriate modifications to allow expired air to come out through the larynx. This is known as fenestration (Table 34-3).

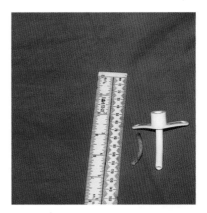

Fig 34-7 The tube from the patient in Fig 34-6; it was changed immediately when suction failed to improve the airway and this large cast of dried secretions was found in the lumen!

Key Point:

Incorrect placement of a tracheostomy tube is a real risk for the inexperienced (Fig 34-8).

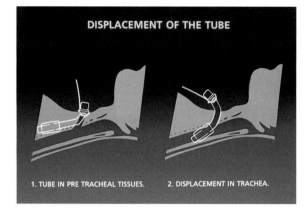

Fig 34-8 Two common ways of misplacing a standard tracheal tube. The misplacement into the pretracheal tissues shown on the left is particularly dangerous and more likely to happen if inserted by the inexperienced.

Table 34-3. Pros and Cons of Different Types of Tracheostomy Tubes

Uncuffed Tubes	Cuffed Tubes
Allow secretions to be inhaled	Prevent aspiration of secretions
Do not touch tracheal wall	Fits against tracheal wall
Suitable for long-term use	Not suitable for long-term use
Air can pass through the vocal cords	Air cannot pass through the vocal cords
Not suitable for ventilation	Suitable for ventialtion

CRICOTHYROIDOTOMY

Crycothyroidotomy or mini-tracheostomy is becoming increasingly popular. Its main value is as an emergency access point to the airway (as above). It is also advocated for airway access to facilitate aspiration of bronchial sections in patients with poor cough—especially those in intensive care. This procedure was popular in the early twentieth century but was discouraged by Chevalier Jackson in the 1920s due to the high incidence of laryngeal stenosis. In current practice it is probably wise to limit cricothyroid access to fairly short periods

Key Point:

Cricothyroidotomy is not a substitute for tracheostomy.

QUINSY

This is an abscess in the peritonsillar region. It is usually due to streptococcal infection and causes severe pain with trismus. Examination shows a grossly asymmetric soft palate with displacement of the uvula away from the side of the quinsy.

Treatment is by aspiration or drainage coupled with high doses of penicillin. Some surgeons practice emergency tonsillectomy for this but the procedure is technically difficult. Following a quinsy, some surgeons recommend interval tonsillectomy (about 6 weeks later). In fact the risk of repeated attacks is not great unless the patient has a history of recurrent tonsillitis or of previous quinsy.

NECK SPACE INFECTIONS

Ludwig's Angina

This is an anaerobic infection of the floor of the mouth and submandibular triangle. The infection encompasses both sides of the mylohyoid muscle causing distension below the mandible and also elevation of the floor of the mouth. This causes the tongue to be displaced upwards with consequent dysphagia and airway blockage. *Treatment* is by drainage and intravenous antibiotics.

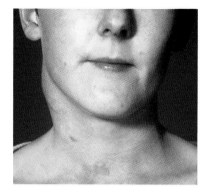

Fig 34-9 A parapharyngeal abscess presenting in the right upper neck in a young man.

Parapharyngeal Abscess

This is usually due to tonsillar infection or occasionally lower jaw dental disease. Swelling is seen in the upper part of the neck behind and below the angle of the mandible (Fig 34-9). Examination of the mouth reveals medial displacement of the tonsil on the affected side only. *Treatment* is by drainage and intravenous antibiotics.

Retropharyngeal Infection

Retropharyngeal infections are uncommon and usually occur in children, especially under 2 years of age. *Treatment* is by drainage. This condition is rare in adults and is usually related to tuberculosis of the cervical vertebrae.

Key Point:
Only the retropharyngeal abscess is drained through the mouth. All other abscesses are drained externally.

LARYNGEAL TRAUMA

This is uncommon but should always be considered in accident departments or intensive care units when dealing with patients with multiple injuries. Look for surgical emphysema of the neck and abnormal crepitus of the laryngeal framework. The voice will be abnormal but patients in this condition are often unconscious. Early intubation and surgical reconstitution are recommended.

FOREIGN BODIES

Both children and adults may be affected. Children will swallow anything but coins are common. Adults usually suffer from food

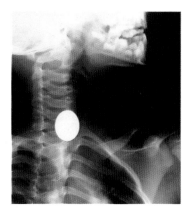

Fig 34-10 A coin in the upper esophagus of a young child. This is one of the commonest foreign bodies seen in children.

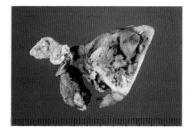

Fig 34-11 This huge piece of pork chop was impacted in the esophagus of a mentally retarded teenager.

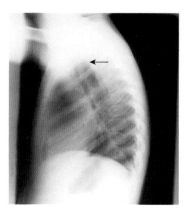

Fig 34-12 A lateral chest X ray showing an intratracheal pin (arrow) that has been inhaled by a child.

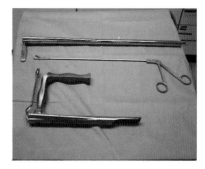

Fig 34-13 Some of the instruments used for rigid endoscopy under general anesthesia, including an esophagoscope above and a pharyngoscope below with biopsy forceps in between.

impaction, eg, bones and badly chewed meat (Figs 34-10, 34-11, and 34-12). This is especially common in edentulous adults who may even swallow their dentures—which are usually not radio-opaque.

Clinical Presentation

The history of clinical symptoms is paramount in deciding the presence or absence of an ingested foreign body. When the patient has clear recall of the ingestion of the item and absolute dysphagia ensues with drooling of saliva , inability to complete the meal, etc., the diagnosis is easy. However, this is not always the case! Pain is almost universal.

Key Points:

1. Fish bones almost always lodge in the tonsils/base of the tongue and are usually not visible with plain X rays.

2. A normal plain X ray does not exclude a foreign body.

3. Always believe the patient.

Examination

Salivary pooling and pain are revealed on palpation of the neck. Radiology may be helpful occasionally but is not critical. Specialized studies may be performed in cases of doubt—either a barium swallow, tomography of the neck, or CT scanning.

Key Point:

The symptoms of foreign body ingestion are more important than specialized investigations.

Treatment

Management in all suspected cases is removal of the foreign body, usually by rigid endoscopy (Fig 34-13).

Index

....